The

ORCHESTRA CONDUCTOR'S

SECRET

to HEALTH & LONG LIFE

Conducting and Other Easy Things to Do to Feel Better,
Keep Fit, Lose Weight, Increase Energy, and Live Longer

DALE L. ANDERSON, MD

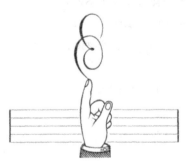

C H R O N I M E D
P U B L I S H I N G

The Orchestra Conductor's Secret to Health & Long Life: Conducting and Other Easy Things to Do to Feel Better, Keep Fit, Lose Weight, Increase Energy, and Live Longer © 1997 by Dale L. Anderson

Library of Congress Cataloging-in-Publication Data
Anderson, Dale, 1933-
The orchestra conductor's secret to health and long life / Dale Anderson.

ISBN 978-1-62045-713-9

Editor: Jeff Braun
Cover Design: Emerson, Wajdowicz Studios Inc./NYC
Text Design: David Enyeart
Figure Drawings by Margo Bock Exsted
Art/Production Manager: Claire Lewis
Printed in the United States of America

Published by Chronimed Publishing
P.O. Box 59032
Minneapolis, MN 55459-9686

10   9   8   7   6   5   4   3   2   1

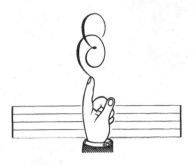

About the Author

Dale L. Anderson, M.D., an assistant clinical professor at the University of Minnesota Medical School, has been a physician for over 38 years and has practiced as a family doctor, a board certified general surgeon, and a board certified emergency physician. His current practice is in the Urgent Care Department of a large Minnesota clinic. Dr. Anderson is a member of the American Medical Association, The American College of Surgeons, the American Association of Therapeutic Humor, and the National Speakers Association. He is past president of the Medical Speakers Association and the Minnesota Speakers Association. He coordinates the Minnesota ACT NOW! Project, which adapts theater art techniques "that play out 'well' on the health stage." He is one of America's leading health "edu-tainers" and conducts seminars internationally through his speaking company, J'ARM, Inc.

To many inspiring patients who over the years have repeatedly demonstrated that we can often choose the right health moves to "magically" elevate the "inner uppers" that raise our spirits and get us high on life.

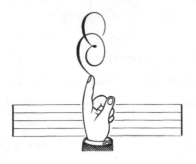

Acknowledgments

A SPECIAL THANKS TO:

Minnesota physician and health care friends and colleagues, and the many hearty and wonderful Minnesota patients and friends who have helped make Minnesota the healthiest state in the nation.

James Reinertsen, M.D., C.E.O. of HealthSystem Minnesota, A. Stuart Hanson, M.D., President of Institute for Research and Education–HealthSystem Minnesota, and Glen D. Nelson, M.D., Vice Chairman of Medtronic, Incorporated—who were instrumental in fostering and promoting the health education program SHAPE. The program has helped add days to the lives of many and life to the days of all who learn and follow its teachings about healthful lifestyles.

Jim Toscano, Vice President and C.O.O., Institute for Research and Education–HealthSystem Minnesota, for encouraging the writing of this book.

The talented friends of the National Speakers Association for setting high platform standards and for inspiring me to strive to achieve their expected quality of performance excellence.

John Pope for his promotional advice and counsel.

Douglas Toft for his editorial and writing expertise.

The dedicated and professional staff of Chronimed Publishing.

And last and most importantly, with much love—to Britta, Ethan, and "The Anderson Clan."

Notice: Consult your health care professional

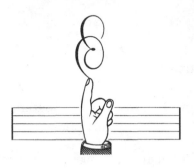

Contents

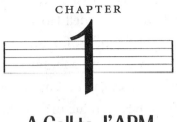

A Call to J'ARM

Where words fail, music speaks.
—Hans Christian Andersen

IT WAS GEORGE, A DELIGHTFUL RETIRED LINE WORKER WHO SAID to me when he was 67 years old, "I know I need more exercise. But with my bad hips, it's painful to jog. I don't like swimming, and I feel self-conscious at the health clubs with all those trim, beautiful, perspiring young women putting the rush on me." (George had a vivid imagination.) He also spoke of the three M's that made him shy away from health clubs: machines, mirrors, and massive muscles.

George recalled as a young man in his 20s that he was "trim and fit as a fiddle." Back then he and his wife did a lot of dancing, and he even worked for a few years as a band director and sang in a barbershop quartet. "Those were the active good old days, Doc, never felt better. Music around me, music within me. Just the memory of those times strikes up the band in my mind."

Profound, I thought, as I listened to George. He brought to mind the words of Oliver Wendell Holmes: "Too many people die with their music in them." Unfortunately, too many people don't even know that they have a fantastic orchestra within— an orchestra for which they can become a masterful conductor.

"How did it feel to be a conductor?" I asked.

George thought for a moment. Then he told me how healthy and happy he felt when he was actively conducting. "You know, it was kind of like jogging—with the arms," he said.

From that simple observation came the word J'ARM— (J)ogging with the (ARM)s. George's reply was the seed for a harvest of health benefits for him, as it can be for you.

Professional conductors have known about the benefits of J'ARMING, even if they didn't use the term. Great symphony orchestra conductors tend to live longer—an average of five years longer, in fact—than the general population. They also are said to be healthier in both mind and body than many others in their age group. In 1980, the Metropolitan Life Insurance Company published the results of a study on the longevity of conductors. Researchers looked at the lifespans of 437 active and former conductors of regional and community orchestras across America. The conclusion: Mortality among symphony conductors was 38 percent below their contemporaries in the general population.

For example, Toscanini died just two months and two days before his ninetieth birthday. Leopold Stokowski lived to be 95. Arthur Fiedler was 85, and Bruno Walter was 86. Even Leonard Bernstein, who died at the relatively young age of 72, beat the odds. "God knows, I should be dead by now," Bernstein remarked a couple of years before his death. "I smoke. I drink. I stay up all night. I'm overcommitted on all fronts. I was told that if I didn't stop smoking, I'd be dead at 35. Well, I beat the rap."

One of the things that helps these people beat the rap is the sheer fun of conducting—making those grand, sweeping motions of the arms surrounded by an ocean of sound. There's a large element of play in conducting. "You can't be serious 24 hours a day. You have to take half-an-hour or an hour a day to be childish," said Vladimir Horowitz. "Conducting is a real sport," noted Aaron Copland. "You can never guarantee what the results are going to be, so there's always an element of chance. That keeps it exciting."

We can't say there is a direct, cause-and-effect relationship between conducting movements and living into one's eighties or nineties. Other factors are probably at work—among them, commitment to a vocation, connection to other people, and a passion for music. (More about these factors in Chapter Six on the "C personality.") Yet the correlation between conducting and the health of these musicians is striking.

Many of us can recall with fond memories times when, as children, we captured something of the excitement these great musicians must feel. At those times we directed music naturally. We threw our arms up in the air and marched around, moving to the music. Some of us even pretended that we were leading a large orchestra as we stood in front of a mirror. Many of us who see a conductor at work have to fight back the urge once again to become like a child and mimic those movements. We'd love to let go and allow our bodies to flow with the music.

J'ARMING gives you the excuse. In this book you get a prescription from a physician to let yourself go, regress a little bit, and at the same time regenerate in both mind and body. You can

lift a baton and become a conductor, band leader, or choir director. You can recapture that excitement, that feeling of being in
control, of moving out of yourself, leaving stress and pain
behind, and connecting spiritually with others. One woman says
she feels a sense of oneness with "nature, God, and the universe."
Some have felt the body lifting, the mind running free. And the
more they J'ARM—jog with the arms—the better they feel.

I encourage everyone to J'ARM. At the end of my speaking
programs, I always include a short J'ARMING session. I pass out
special J'ARM sticks (chopsticks, a symbol of healthful eating
habits) and play upbeat, lively songs to which the audience and
I J'ARM. Audiences always get their arms moving to the music.
Soon they are laughing, marching, and conducting themselves
in a healthy, carefree manner, enjoying themselves in a way that
many haven't experienced in years.

J'ARMING is a crowd pleaser, but it isn't just something to do
for amusement. J'ARMING really does yield health benefits. This
result will become clear as we understand the physical, physiological, and psychological benefits of using the arms to conduct
our "inner music." Tune in!

Your amazing arms

Your arms are an underused source of energy, fitness, and
health. By exercising your arms you reap these benefits:
- Better posture
- Improved muscle strength and flexibility
- A gentle back and shoulder massage
- A suppressed appetite (if you exercise before eating)
- Weight reduction
- A "wash" for your brain that removes distractions

- A positive attitude and readiness for laughter
- A reduction of your physiological and mental ages

You'll be reading more about these benefits throughout this book.

The thought of regular arm exercising may sound painful. Yet our arms are much stronger than many people realize and soon build stamina. Just think about the times we "overdo" their usage. Despite the temporary aches and pains from a day of raking, painting, shoveling, or gardening, most of us feel invigorated from working out our arms.

A fun and effective way to exercise your arms is to "jog" your arms to happy, invigorating music. When you J'ARM, you enjoy the exercise's advantages: no expensive equipment or wardrobe, no weather woes, no special positions. There's no impact of hip, knees, or feet, and no potholes or dogs to contend with. J'ARMING does not require you to join the ranks of the sleek people sweating it out on rowing machines. You can do it at home on your own schedule and it's easy, fun, and effective.

J'ARMing as a form of exercise

Exercise: why does it sometimes sound like a four-letter word? We've heard about its benefits countless times. Yet many people would rather undergo a root canal than keep up a regular exercise program. They dismiss the idea with a quip: For them, exercise is walking to the corner tavern and lifting a heavy mug of "lite" beer, stepping over the bathroom scale each morning, running up a bill, jumping to conclusions, or climbing the walls.

One woman described a novel exercise program, which was going home after a hard day's work, running a bathtub full of hot water, and climbing in to relax the day's cares away. Then when she started feeling a little guilty about her inactivity, she would pull the plug and fight the current.

Please don't misunderstand: I'm not against relaxation. In fact, I advocate a daily time for de-stressing. It's just that relaxation and exercise can go together. They don't have to be at odds with each other.

Study after study tells us we need to keep moving. But for many of us these studies are more a threat than an encouragement. Often they put too much stress on athletic prowess. They make it seem that reaping health benefits requires a lot of hard work. As one of my patients put it, "I could never become a Jockasauraus Rex." Who needs it? Who has time?

My patients certainly exercise, particularly the "vintage patients" I call VPS. And most now have time. All I need to do is sell them on the benefits of exercise and persuade them of the unique advantages of J'ARMING.

By now it's well known that regular exercise is associated with a long list of health benefits. Among them are strengthened and flexible muscles, improved heart and lung efficiency, and weight control. Reminded of this fact, most of the people I talk to readily admit they could profit from increased activity. At the same time, many of them press me with a further question: Why choose J'ARMING over other forms of exercise? What's the big deal about J'ARMING anyway?

My response, in a nutshell, is that J'ARMING brings the whole person into play. J'ARMING fully involves you on the physical, mental, and emotional levels, all at once. In addition, there's the presence of music. Great music, like all great art, can do more than merely occupy your mind; it can refine and expand your thoughts as well. Even popular songs, big band music, and the old "standards" can produce something of the same effect. Songs can help you recall a pleasant past event because music is often associated with those "good feeling times." This fact is especially true when you choose songs with lyrics that plant positive thoughts and images in your mind. When you J'ARM you can sing those lyrics, which increases the aerobic effect of J'ARMING because you use up more oxygen.

In short, J'ARMING is a multisensory experience. Touch, hearing, sight, movement, and sense of balance all come into play. There's the sound of the music and the feel of the baton in your hand. And if you stand when you J'ARM, the motion of your arms induces you to assume a more erect posture, one that preserves a healthful arch in the lower part of your back and encourages upper back flexibility. Many people can get the same effect even if they sit while J'ARMING

It's true that much aerobic dance exercise is done to music, but that music is often little more than drums with a heavy backbeat and electric bass, booming away in the background at one monotonous volume level. When you J'ARM, the music comes to the forefront. And it can be quality music, which I define simply as any music that you enjoy. The pleasure provides a built-in incentive to exercise.

While J'ARMING is simple to do, its simplicity is deceptive. This form of exercise brings into play a variety of physical and mental processes. It "orchestrates" our bodies and minds, helping them work together for an optimal effect—helping you tune in and tune up.

There are many ways to get good arm exercise, but for me, J'ARMING, pretending I'm a great symphony or choral conductor, is one of the easiest and most fun.

J'ARMing is smart exercise

Every time we exercise our arms, our brains say "thank you" just a little bit more emphatically than they do when we exercise our legs. Because the arms share a main artery with the brain, exercising the arms also increases the flow of blood to the brain. (By moving our arms, we improve blood circulation to the brain.)

Why this happens becomes clear when we look at some simple anatomy. Start with the aorta, the the great artery that carries blood from the heart for distribution throughout the body. The first vessel off the arch of the aorta is called the brachiocephalic trunk. It divides into two vessels of nearly equal size: the carotid that carries blood to the head, and the subclavian that carries blood to the arm. When one uses the arms they demand a greater blood supply from the heart, and half of the blood called for by the arms is diverted to the head. The head thereby enjoys enhanced nutrition and oxygen supply.

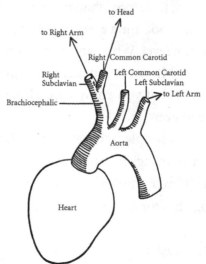

Some anthropologists postulate that this connection is one reason we as humans evolved a much larger brain than other animals. More specifically, the human opposable thumb, along with well-developed arms and hands, made activities possible that hoofs, fins, claws, and other "hands" could not achieve. The more the thumbs and hands were used, the more blood went to the brain, and the larger the brain became. And as their brains grew, humans discovered more ways to use their hands.

Such a development was not accomplished overnight. The Bible tells us that God created human kind on the sixth day. Yet that "day" may have occurred over millions of years. In any case, the abundant flow of blood that carried oxygen and nutrition to the head provided the best environment for developing the brain.

Does this mean that people who exercise their arms may be more intelligent than those who don't? I won't give you a definitive answer to that one, other than my opinion that people who J'ARM are the smartest of all. As a white-haired physician with more than forty years of experience caring for patients, I'm convinced that J'ARMING can add days to your life and life to your days. I often say, only half kidding, that if you want to clear your head, move your arms and learn to J'ARM.

What this book includes

In this book, you'll learn the many benefits of J'ARMING and how to become what I call a "J'ARMING Lady" or a "Prince J'ARMING." As you read, keep in mind that this is not a music book, and that J'ARMING requires no musical aptitude. You won't need to read any textbooks on conducting or take a music appreciation course. J'ARMING is first and foremost a form of exercise that emphasizes using the arms.

Chapter Two, "What J'ARMING Can Do for You," explains some of the possible benefits of J'ARMING. These include raising your endorphin level, improving heart-lung efficiency, regulating your weight, improving your posture, and more.

Chapter Three, "How to J'ARM" offers instructions for J'ARM-ING. You'll begin by learning about selecting music to J'ARM by, tools of the J'ARMING trade, and when and where you can J'ARM. Then follows a basic, intermediate, and advanced course in J'ARMING along with some supplemental exercises and ways to round out your J'ARMING program.

Chapter Four, "J'ARMING and the New Science of Health," relates J'ARMING to a relatively new field called psychoneuroimmunology (PNI). Even though this field has a long, complicated name, its focus is quite down to earth: the role of positive thoughts and emotions in creating and sustaining health.

Chapter Five, "How to Extend the Benefits of J'ARMING—Becoming a C Personality," puts J'ARMING in the larger context of overall wellness. In its most profound meaning, staying healthy means taking into account mental, emotional, and social factors. Besides conditioning our bodies, we can condition our minds and spirits as well. That involves the "five C's"—being conditioned, connected, challenged, committed, and controlled. Together they make up an approach to life that typifies the "C personality."

Chapter Six, "You're a J'ARMER," reviews the key principles of this book and sends you on your way to a lifetime of improved health.

At the end of this book you'll find some suggestions for music to J'ARM by, along with ideas for further reading about how the mind, emotions, and body can work together for better health.

In a previous book, *Act Now* (Chronimed Publishing), I discuss many ways that you can "get your act together" to set the stage for dramatic changes in your life and physiology. All performing artists, including orchestra conductors, know that to be "on a roll," they need to be "in the role." Your role is to tune into yourself, and "play your high notes."

Psychoneuroimmunology, which includes the study of endorphins and related healthy chemistries, now shows that inner chemistry can be acted on and conducted on. This makes it all the more tragic that so many people don't understand that they have music within themselves—that they can learn to "play up."

What J'ARMing Can Do for You

Disease is not only suffering, but also the body fighting to restore itself to normal—a sort of healing force within.

—Hippocrates

YOU CAN REAP THE MOST BENEFITS FROM J'ARMING, LIKE ANY other exercise program, by getting started as early as possible. Yet one fear holds many people back—the possibility of "overdoing it." People who come to my office with body stiffness and aches and pains often express this fear. What they could say instead is, "I underdo so much that when I do do, I often end up feeling like I overdid!" Rarely do people complain that they are out-of-shape couch potatoes or deconditioned chair jockeys. They usually don't tell me they need to become revitalized. Often they don't see that they can build up some cardiorespiratory and muscular "reserve" to handle the normal stress and strains of a lifestyle that is enjoyable and challenging.

One of my patients, Margie, came to the office complaining of many aches and pains. You name the trouble spot—Margie had it. She had worked most of her life at a desk job and devoted the weekends to spectator entertainment and household chores. Margie left exercise to the kids. Her request was, "Fix me, Doc."

Sorry, Margie, I said to myself. Instead, you have the opportunity to fix yourself. First you'll change your posture. Then you'll start an exercise program and become a J'ARMER. Start the music!

I asked Margie if she had heard the expression, "Use it or lose it."

"Yes, I've heard it many times," she said.

"Well, you lost it," I replied. "But you can find it again with simple exercise. First understand the benefits of exercise in general and J'ARMING in particular."

For Margie, as for most of us, these can include:
- Improving heart-lung efficiency
- Improving flexibility and balance
- Strengthening muscles
- Raising the level of brain chemicals known as endorphins
- Regulating weight
- Improving posture
- Higher self-esteem

Improve your heart-lung efficiency

For the heart and lungs to be as healthy as they can be, they need the conditioning that results from periodically raising the pulse rate a bit. This conditioning helps the heart and lungs grow stronger.

There are many formulas for finding an ideal heart rate (pulse) for exercise. The most familiar is 220 minus your age times 0.7. For example, if you are 54, your ideal pulse rate during exercise would be around 116. (220 minus 54 equals 166; 166 times 0.7 equals about 116.) Even so, you don't have to keep your heart rate at this level every time you exercise.

Several years ago we were told that exercise benefitted us fully only if we raised the target heart rate for 20 to 30 minutes, three to four times a week. Now we know that lower exercise heart rates are also beneficial. Indeed, any body movement that stretches us, strengthens our muscles, or even slightly raises our heart rate and deepens breathing is useful.

I asked Margie to exercise until her heart rate was 110 and to maintain that, if possible, for 20 minutes. Over a period of months, her heart-lung efficiency improved, and she had to add more physical effort to hit the target heart rate during exercise. At the same time, Margie found it easier to do the level of exercise she had once found difficult.

In engineering terms, Margie's heart-lung machinery was becoming more efficient. She required less effort for tasks such as climbing stairs, hauling groceries, or playing with children.

Improve your flexibility and balance

When she first came to see me, Margie moved in jerky, stiff movements. She looked as if she were about to break. That her tissues were tight and stiff was obvious to anyone who looked at her. What's more, Margie appeared fearful of losing her balance.

Such are the ravaging results of a deconditioned, sedentary lifestyle. All the soft connective tissue in the muscles, tendons, and ligaments become like tight rubber bands or hardened rubber cement spilled about the joints. When the joints aren't stretched, they move poorly. In addition, the balancing nerves (called proprioceptors) wither, or atrophy, from underuse.

Fortunately, the tight tissues, just like tight rubber bands, can be stretched and become more flexible. A simple exercise, the "relaxing stretch," loosens any area of tightness. I recommend using this stretch in conjunction with J'ARMING. You'll find instructions for the relaxing stretch on page 55.

Strengthen your muscles

Using a muscle makes that muscle stronger. A strong muscle does any work with greater ease. If a muscle is not used, it loses its strength rapidly. In fact, one week of inactivity causes a muscle to lose 15 to 20 percent of its strength (work capacity).

The muscle groups that I see older people lose most frequently are the upper arm and shoulder group and the upper leg-groin muscle group. We use the upper leg and groin muscles to sit down on a chair and raise ourselves up again. These muscles also assist in walking.

Muscle weakness, especially the inability to get up from a chair, is a major cause of nursing home admissions. I told Margie the story of my Aunt Thelma, who at age 82 lived alone and led a sedentary life. She sat to drive her car. She sat to visit with friends and relatives. She sat to watch television and read. Thelma rarely used her "get up and go" muscles. To get out of a chair, Thelma needed to push herself up with her arms or ask someone for a "pull me up." In short, she sat… and sat… and sat.

Eventually, Aunt Thelma developed weak muscles in her upper leg and groin, and had a hard time rising from a sitting position. Then she got the flu and pneumonia and spent two weeks in bed. She recovered, but after the illness she had lost so much muscle strength—20 to 40 percent of her reserve—that she never walked alone again.

Thelma didn't drive again, either. Instead, she sat continuously until someone helped her up to walk. Because she couldn't get up to take care of herself, Thelma entered a nursing home. There she spent most of her time in bed, growing progressively weaker. You can well guess the ending of this story.

All this trouble was unnecessary. If Thelma had developed strong muscles before her illness, she would have had sufficient reserve to resume full functioning afterward and could have continued an active, independent life.

J'ARMING strengthens muscles, especially in the upper body. Just the simple weight of the arm and the baton is sufficient to build muscle endurance. Later on, you may want to add "up and down" or "in and out of the chair" routines to exercise the upper leg-groin muscle group. Doing so greatly decreases your risk of becoming another Aunt Thelma.

Raise your endorphin level

As mentioned earlier, a new branch of science called psychoneuroimmunology (PNI) is devoted to studying body chemistries. Lately certain chemicals have gained attention, particularly in the lay press. I call these our "inner uppers," the endorphins, seemingly magic chemicals from the "pharmacy within." Produced in the brain and other tissues, they have a structure almost identical to synthetic or plant-derived injectable morphine. That means endorphins can deliver the kind of pain relief and euphoria associated with morphine.

Endorphins have been known to us for only about twenty years, but the idea that certain substances in the body are associated with specific moods and feelings is an ancient one. For centuries, people were classified according to temperament.

According to this viewpoint, temperament was determined by which fluids (humors) dominated the body. Anger denoted too much bile in the system; passivity meant too much phlegm.

Like the practice of blood-letting and other unscientific methods of healing, the theory of bodily humors has fallen well out of favor. Yet it's possible that the basic idea behind this theory has some merit. Current brain research emphasizes the role of certain substances in producing emotion.

The brain at work

What would you see if you could look inside a brain at work? The answer to this question is complex, but in essence you'd see a lot of fireworks—millions of tiny reactions. Neurons, or nerve cells, are the building blocks of the brain and spinal cord. These cells fire off electrical charges and chemicals to other nerve cells and muscles, and each charge or chemical has a specific effect.

In essence, these charges and chemicals make up the "messages" the nervous system sends to the rest of the body, and those messages regulate our thoughts and moods. As brain researcher Robert Ornstein puts it, such chemicals are "words" the body uses to communicate. The endorphins are one group of these nerve chemicals.

How endorphins were discovered

Ironically enough, we first found out about endorphins by studying a flower—the poppy. Humans have used poppy juice, also known as opium, for thousands of years to reduce pain and stimulate pleasure. Morphine is the main active ingredient in opium, and it's still used to treat severe pain.

In the early 1970s, however, some scientists wondered why

this substance from a plant has such a powerful effect on human beings. The answer, they guessed, is that the brain produces its own form of opiates—its own "internal morphine."

What followed was a worldwide race, of sorts, to find these natural opiates. Two researchers from the University of Aberdeen in Scotland were the first to do so, in 1975. Since then, other internally produced opiates have been discovered in the human body, and there may be many more. What an exciting area of research! And there are sure to be more new developments.

The power of endorphins

Back to the endorphins. These internally-produced chemicals attach to cells at the same sites as injectable morphine and therefore affect us much as injectable morphine does. Endorphins can prevent certain other brain cells from transmitting impulses, giving endorphins the power to block pain and produce feelings of euphoria.

These effects make endorphins crucial ingredients in our "pharmacy within." That internal pharmacy has several advantages over the drugs you buy from a drugstore. For one, endorphins are free. The adverse side effects of endorphins are minimal or nonexistent. What's more, endorphins made inside the body are anywhere from 200 to 2,000 times more potent than injectable morphine.

One of the reasons many people become addicted to morphine-type substances is that they develop euphoria, a feeling of mental well-being. The more they use injectable morphine, however, the more they turn off the production of their own bodily morphine (endorphins).

After the addict stops using morphine or one of the morphine derivatives, it takes a long time for the body to recover its ideal endorphin-raising capabilities.

It is these gifts from our internal pharmacy—the endorphins—that create a feeling of elation, a euphoria that gets us "high on life." Though we don't understand exactly how they work, we have strong evidence that endorphins and their healthy psychoneuroimmune (PNI) chemical "cousins" are raised by a wide range of activities. Among them are laughter, positive imaging, satisfying relationships, setting and reaching goals, parties, meaningful rituals, and—yes—just believing that something will do us good. Another strategy for raising endorphins is regular exercise such as J'ARMING

The endorphins and PNI chemicals are lowered in certain people—those who have poor posture, who have poor physical conditioning, or who are deficient in the three S's of stamina, strength, and stretching. People with chronic pain or stress may start to use up some of their endorphin stores, and those who depend regularly on pain-relieving medications may turn off their endorphin production.

The benefits associated with raising the endorphins include pain relief, tension relief, strengthening the immune system, and even improved relationships.

Endorphins and pain relief

Norman Cousins, in his book *Anatomy of an Illness*, got many people thinking about the importance of mental attitude in control of pain. He stated that if he could laugh for 10 minutes he would be pain free for two hours. It's quite possible that Cousins' endorphin level was raised during these periods of happy thoughts and laughter.

Endorphins and tension relief

Once the endorphins are raised, the muscles become more relaxed and tensions are eased. Maybe you've had the experience of carrying a piece of heavy furniture with a friend when one of you said something funny. You probably had to put the object down because the muscles were so "weak." This weakness was probably the relaxation response triggered by your laughter, which stimulated endorphin production..

Endorphins and related chemicals can also be raised merely by imagining that a medication or a treatment works. This technique can sometimes be used to relieve muscular tension, headaches, and back pain. Imagine tension flowing out of your body, and let the endorphins do the rest. This is an example of pos"I"tive thinking—using happy thoughts to promote health.

Not only can physical pain be reduced by raising endorphins—often a reduction in mental and emotional pain comes as well. When the endorphins rise, the euphoric state that occurs does not permit depression, anger, or fear. A measurable increase in serum endorphins has great potential for "clearing the mind," clearing a mental space for positive emotions.

Endorphins and the immune system

When the endorphins are elevated, the immune system also functions better. People who raise their endorphin levels usually have greater numbers of t-cells, n-cells, and gamma globulins. All of these internal substances effectively fight bacteria and viruses. Many cancer specialists believe that raising endorphin levels is an important factor in the survival rate of their patients. It appears that stimulating the endorphins and related chemicals correlates with a longer and healthier life.

Endorphins and the social pleasures

Many other benefits accompany increased endorphins. People who know how to raise endorphin levels, not only in themselves but also in others, are often popular, physically attractive, and report more confidence, creativity, courage, and control over their lives than their endorphin-poor peers. A lifestyle full of endorphin-raising activities may even be associated with higher incomes. (We can genuinely say raising endorphins "makes cents.") Individuals who can raise and keep endorphin levels high have been shown to relate better to themselves, their families and friends, and with people in general.

We can't say there's a direct cause-effect relationship between raised endorphins and all the social, physical, and emotional benefits just named. In other words, raising your endorphin level won't guarantee you higher income, better relationships, creativity, all the rest. So far all we can say is that such benefits are associated with raised endorphin levels—not caused by those endorphin levels. Yet that association is strong enough to merit serious attention.

J'ARMING includes a number of activities that stimulate endorphin production—exercise, laughter, positive attitudes, music, and even creative visualization.

When you J'ARM, you're filling a powerful prescription from your pharmacy within.

Regulate your weight

After many years of medical practice, I've heard and seen the results of hundreds of "quick-fix" diets. Most of these schemes have been touted by self-made experts who make outlandish, unscientific claims. And many of the folks who followed the easy, magic formulas had unrealistic expectations. Often they were rewarded with disappointment and failure. Some even became ill.

Still we see a new diet book or a new dietary supplement or aid every few months. These new diet fads hang on for a short time—until the dieters become discouraged—and then we wait for the next diet "secret" to be revealed.

Our society is constantly getting on and off diets. As a result, our collective weight goes down and up, down and up, up, and down and eventually up, up, up. This method of dieting has been called the yo-yo or roller coaster diet cycle. I call it the "Rhythm Method of Girth Control."

The Rhythm Method has not, will not, and cannot work. The scientific reasons it can't work are documented in the dietary advice and literature of the American Heart Association, American Diabetes Association, and the American Cancer Society. These prestigious organizations, along with recognized nutrition experts, generally agree on how to lose weight safely. They recommend similar principles:

- A modest restriction in calories
- An increase in use of fiber (fruits, vegetables, and grains)
- A reduction of the total fat calories in our diets to 30 percent or less, with particular attention to lowering saturated fats from animal products and tropical oils.
- An increase of calories from carbohydrates to 55 percent or more of total calories consumed.

In addition, reputable experts emphasize exercise as a critical, if not the most important ingredient, in a successful weight reduction plan. This is where J'ARMING enters the picture.

I tell my patients that dieting can be "a piece of cake." It doesn't need to be difficult if we just "chip" away, little by little, until we eventually have the body weight (within genetic reason) that is our goal.

Diaita is the Greek word from which our word diet derives. When I ask patients to guess the meaning of *diaita*, I usually get answers like hardship, deprivation, struggle, torture. When they look the word up in a dictionary, they're surprised to find that it means "way of life."

Let's look at the simple arithmetic behind a dieting way of life. A pound of fat has 3,500 calories. Therefore, to lose a pound of fat we must consume 3,500 fewer calories or burn up 3,500 calories through exercise. We can, of course, combine the two and take in fewer calories as we burn up more.

If you cut just 10 calories each day from your diet, you eliminate 3,650 calories a year—more than a pound of fat. What is 10 calories? One peanut. Half a potato chip. One-fourth of a pat of butter. Letting go of these calories can be easy. Add moderate exercise, and it becomes even easier. If you climb 20 steps a day (one flight) you burn 10 calories. Do this every day and you'll burn 3,650 calories over a year. Again, that's more than a pound of fat. Do both and lose two pounds a year. Simple lifestyle changes can result in significant health benefits.

One overweight man who came to see me drank five cans of sugared soft drink per day. That's about 160 calories per can. If he could make one of those cans a diet soft drink (one calorie), he could practically eliminate 160 calories per day. Over the period of one year, that equals a reduction of over 58,000 calories—about 16 pounds. And what if he switched all five cans to diet soft drink? Then the potential weight loss jumps to about 80 pounds per year. Imagine that kind of weight loss, just from changing one simple habit.

Similarly, if you switch from a glass of 2 percent milk to a glass of 3 percent milk, you eliminate 30 calories. At one glass per day, that's a loss of nearly three pounds per year. And going from one glass of 3 percent milk to a glass of skim milk takes ninety calories a day out of the diet—a potential weight loss of nine pounds per year. As another example, say that you eat chocolate cake several times per week. Each piece of chocolate cake with chocolate icing contains about 350 calories. Cut out one piece of chocolate cake per week and you could lose seven pounds per year.

To reinforce the idea of a gradual change in diet, think of it as similar to reducing the heat in your home by turning down the thermostat on your furnace just one degree at a time. For example, calories from fat commonly make up 40 to 50 percent of an American's diet. Reducing this to 20 or 30 percent overnight is much too steep a change for anyone. That would be like asking people who've kept their thermostats at 80 degrees for years to immediately turn them back to 68 degrees—a strategy that's likely to fail.

However, there's a greater chance of success when people decrease the thermostat setting gradually—say, one or two degrees each week—until they reach 68 degrees. In terms of eating, this means gradually reducing calorie or fat intake as described above. Remember, even cutting 10 calories a day can add up to big results.

When choosing where to cut down on calories, remember that all calories are not created equal. Fats in the diet are efficiently placed into fat tissue storage. Very little body fuel is needed to move fat from the blood and store it in fat cells. On the other hand, calories that come from carbohydrates need to be converted to fat before they can be stored in fat cells. This conversion of carbohydrate to fat for storage is relatively inefficient. In fact, nearly 25 percent of calories from carbohydrates are burned in this conversion.

So, nearly all the fat in our diet is easily stored as fat, while only 75 percent of excess carbohydrates enter fat storage. Couple this with another fact: One gram of fat contains nine calories, while one gram of carbohydrate contains only four calories. It's easy to understand why nutritionists often say "fat goes to fat," or, "the fat you eat is the fat you wear."

In addition to suggesting that people eliminate as much fat as possible from their diets, I also tell them about another relatively painless way to cut calories: Look at the calories that come from beverages. It's easy to forget that many beverages contain calories we can easily do without.

One simple but powerful dieting strategy for adults is to eliminate all beverages that contain calories (except an occasional alcoholic beverage). Even a glass of skim milk contains about 90 calories. Adults can cut out those calories by reducing or eliminating the milk they drink. Yes! Switch to water with your meals, and get your calcium from calcium supplement pills or by chewing antacids like TUMS or Titralac. Both are rich sources of this nutrient.

One major cause of our overweight population is that we've been oversold on the virtues of fruit juices. I especially disagree with pushing fruit juices on overweight school children under the guise that it's good for them. For example, drinking one four-ounce glass of fruit juice (about 60 calories) per day can add up to six pounds a year. Yet many well-intentioned, health-conscious people drink glass after glass of fruit juice. Better to eat the fruit, ingest fewer calories, get the extra roughage, and painlessly peel off "juicy" fat.

In summary, cut out the excessive calories in the diet that come from sugared soft drinks and fruit beverages. If you're worried about getting enough vitamin C, then take a one-a-day vitamin with mineral supplement.

I'm for any health supplement however that someone thinks will help—provided it does no harm and is not excessively expensive. I warn people, however, to avoid the mega-dose vitamin and mineral fads. Avoid nutrition supplements, often sold by acquaintances involved in a pyramid selling program. Such schemes, for the most part, result in wealthy acquaintances and expensive urine.

The most successful new diets concentrate on these two areas: cutting down on fat, and moderating the amount of calories consumed in beverages. Together with pleasurable exercise, these can become a way of life. J'ARMING, along with modest but steady reduction in calories, easily fills the bill.

As a form of regular exercise, J'ARMING can help you lose weight in several ways:

KEEPING YOU FROM EATING. It's pretty hard to hit the mouth when your hands and arms are busy directing music. Forks or spoons are unprofessional batons for a conductor of your caliber. By the way, I've been asked if it's OK to use a baton to eat. My answer is yes: eat all you want from your baton, provided you use just one and you don't sharpen it to a point.

SUPPRESSING YOUR APPETITE. You'll feel less hungry after J'ARM-ING, probably because the exercise has raised your endorphins, thus decreasing the urge to eat. (Exercise also suppresses the urge to smoke—an urge labeled by the surgeon general as the greatest American health problem.)

BURNING CALORIES. The number of calories you burn while J'ARMING depends on how hard you are directing and how many parts of your body are involved. Obviously, the more vigorous conductor will burn more calories and fat. Keep in mind that for a 130-pound person, a mile walk or jog burns about 100 calories. A lighter person burns slightly less, and a heavier person slightly more. J'ARMING, I believe, is at least as vigorous as walking. Please—don't give up the enjoyable exercise you are now doing. Instead, add J'ARMING to get some added health benefits.

CONTINUING TO BURN CALORIES FOR SEVERAL HOURS AFTER EXERCISE. During exercise the body furnaces are stoked up, and the body's metabolic rate (the speed at which calories are burned) is elevated. The increased metabolic rate remains for several hours after exercise. So a special dividend of any exercise is that we continue to burn calories even after we stop.

USING MUSCLES TO BURN CALORIES. Muscles require more calories than fatty tissue. As you become better conditioned, you will add muscle bulk: the percentage of body fat is reduced, and the percentage of healthy, strong muscle tissue is increased. Muscle tissue has a higher metabolic rate than other tissue. Consequently, if you develop stronger muscles, you can consume a few more calories and still not gain weight. The upper body is often not exercised very much in our modern-day, sedentary lifestyle. That's where J'ARMING comes in. As the college kids say when the biceps start to bulge, you'll look "awesome" in your tee shirt, and other people will begin to take notice.

IMPROVING POSTURE. It takes more effort to sit up or stand straight. Sitting and standing in good posture burns ten additional calories each hour. That alone is a potential weight loss of 10 to 15 pounds per year! J'ARMING automatically places most people in a more erect posture.

This point is so important that it deserves more detail.

Improve your posture

In high school, Tom was looked upon as the all-American boy. Now a middle-aged lawyer, he came into the office one day at the urging of his family. He was starting to look like a LOM (little old man). Indeed, Tom looked substantially older than his fifty-five years. He sat stooped forward, with rounded lower back, humped upper back, forward-jutting chin, and rolled shoulders.

Tom looked at himself in the mirror one day and "got the picture." Age was fast taking its toll. And, as often happens, his thoughts followed his body messages. Tom became convinced he was beginning to feel old as well as look old. Yes, the LOM body posture had started to convince his brain that it was all down hill from here. Tom wondered if he was getting osteoporosis. He'd seen a magazine advertisement with a photograph of a LOL (yup, little old lady) who was urged to buy an expensive calcium supplement. The message was clear: Stooped posture is the result of calcium deficit.

You've probably seen that advertisement yourself, with the LOL all hunched forward. Meanwhile her statuesque young daughter says, "If only mother had known about the 'magic' calcium preparation, she wouldn't have developed her osteoporosis problem." Nonsense. The LOL may have problems with osteoporosis, but her humped, bent look is probably caused by a lifetime of poor posture. The woman in the advertisement lost her flexibility because of poor sitting and sleeping posture habits.

It's a common story. Once many people leave high school, they start to lose their youthful mobility—especially the ability to arch the back. Gone are the days of the solar clothes drier— the sun—when we had to arch the back to hang up the laundry on the clothes line. After leaving school, the LOL in the advertisement probably went to work sitting at a desk or bending over a table or counter. Later she may have married and bent forward to do household chores or lift babies from the crib. She probably slouched while holding the children or relaxing from housework. All these things contributed to poor posture.

For many years, the medical profession and "old wives' tales" told us not to put a backward arch in the lower back (called the lumbar lordodic curve). We believed this kind of arching would result in future back problems. Only ten years ago, in fact, I and many other physicians were "arch enemies" of the back. We told people not to arch the back and not to sleep on their stomachs. Instead, we encouraged them to flatten the lower back.

Today our advice has turned around 180 degrees. Now we're giving people arching exercises to help regenerate bad backs. I give most of my patients back-arching exercises and tell them it's OK to sleep on their stomachs. For many people, I believe, sleeping on the side is far more likely to be detrimental than sleeping on the stomach.

I told Tom not to worry about becoming like the LOL in the ad. I knew he could regain much of the youthfulness of his back—not to mention his body and mind—if he would start a back-arching and stretching program and launch an all-out effort to change his posture habits.

J'ARMING can help you make that change. When people start moving their arms to music, they often find themselves sitting or standing in an erect posture—even if they didn't consciously intend to do so. J'ARMING is one of several activities (including laughing) that naturally induce you to assume a healthful posture. We'll explore this in more detail as we go over the "how-to's" of J'ARMING.

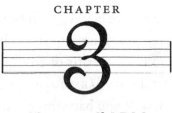

CHAPTER

How to J'ARM

One ought, every day at least, to hear a little song,
read a good poem, see a fine picture, and if it were possible,
to speak a few reasonable words.

—Goethe

"IF I HAD ONLY KNOWN HOW MUCH J'ARMING COULD RELIEVE MY pain, ease my mental tensions, help me lose weight, and feel so good," said Ron, "I would have started J'ARMING many years ago."

Ron became so enthusiastic about teaching the self-steward-ship of good health that he developed a "healthy pleasure" university at his "Over 55" condominium complex. Ron tells his students that to get a J'ARM major, one needs to take Basic J'ARM, Intermediate J'ARM, and an Advanced J'ARM Honors course. This chapter offers more details on each stage of the J'ARMING curriculum.

First, some preliminary matters. These include things to remember before you get started, the role of music, tools of the trade, and when and where to J'ARM.

Before you get started

You've heard this advice before, but it bears repeating: Before beginning any exercise program, consult your physician. In particular, people who have bursitis or trouble rotating the arms and shoulders should start J'ARMING gradually.

Here's a quick test: If you have trouble washing windows or reaching the top shelves in your kitchen, then start J'ARMING slowly. Also remember that you can J'ARM without raising your arms high or separating them widely. Again, be sure to start slowly.

A primary rule of J'ARMING—or any other exercise—is to listen to any signals that your body is experiencing pain. A slight pain you experience only while exercising can be a "good pain" if it is associated with movements. Such pains can mean that you're using some muscles you haven't used in a while, or that you're using muscles in a new way.

Some people experience an achy pain on the day after exercise—a pain that is made worse with muscle use. This means the muscle has been slightly overused and may be an indication to go slow (but still keep going). If pain persists, however, discontinue the exercise and consult your physician. Chances are you will only need to refrain from a particular movement and can still J'ARM safely.

This chapter offers a number of suggestions for J'ARMING. But keep in mind that these are suggestions. There really are no hard and fast rules for J'ARMING. This is an art, not a science. Your J'ARMING technique can be as unique as your fingerprint. Just as each conductor has a different style, so will each person have a different style of J'ARMING.

Music for J'ARMing

Sometimes as I wrote this book, I felt frustrated. I wanted to find a way to lift myself off the printed page and sit with you face-to-face, as I do with the people who come to see me. In this chapter, particularly, I'd like to be able to enter your home. If I could, I'd turn on beautiful, happy music as the background to your reading. Since I can't do this, I suggest that if at all possible, you turn on the most positive, uplifting music you can find and listen to it as you continue reading.

Think for a moment what life would be like without music: no singing your favorite tunes; talk-only radio stations; no concerts; celebrations without songs like *"Happy Birthday," "I Love You Truly,"* and *"Santa Claus Is Coming to Town."* To most of us, life without music is unthinkable.

Music can promote health and serenity. This wisdom is something that human beings have known for centuries. According to Robert Ornstein and David Sobel, the oldest known medical document is a papyrus referring to incantations used in healing the sick. And 2,500 years ago, the philosopher Pythagoras maintained that singing and playing an instrument every day could purge negative emotions such as worry, sorrow, and fear.

To the ancient Greeks, Apollo was the god of both medicine and music.

Greek myths also recount the legend of Orpheus, who used music to charm living creatures. These stories tell us Orpheus played such lovely music on his lyre that animals, trees, and stones followed him. Even rivers stopped flowing in the wake of his music.

Today we know such accounts are not literally true. Yet

modern science indicates that the myths may point to a core of truth. Dorothy Retallack, a researcher in California, studied the effects of music on the life of plants.

She put a variety of plants in chambers with carefully controlled temperature and humidity, then piped in various kinds of music. Judged by their angle of growth and the abundance of their flowers, the plants showed a special fondness for Bach and other Baroque composers. Some of them, in fact, reached out almost as if to embrace the music, turning toward the loudspeakers at 60-degree angles.

Dr. Georgi Lazanov, a Bulgarian psychiatrist, used music as part of a rapid learning program he helped develop in the mid-1960s. While listening to classical music, his students did relaxation exercises, closed their eyes, and listened to an instructor recite French phrases and translations in different voice intonations and rhythms. After the initial session, the students took a test to see how how much they'd learned. The class average was 97 percent, meaning that most of the students learned 1,000 words that day—about half the working vocabulary of a language.

What's more, Dr. Lazanov's students experienced benefits that no one anticipated. Not only did their learning become more rapid and efficient, many reported they felt more relaxed and centered. Tensions, stress, headaches, and other pains seemed to decrease or disappear. Their physiological measurements seemed to back up these reports. It was common for students to experience lower blood pressure and muscle tension, as well as a slower pulse and breathing rhythm.

After that first experiment, organizations across the world began researching and applying Dr. Lazanov's methods under names like "accelerated learning" and "superlearning." As these researchers discovered, our bodies respond to music's rhythms. Music with 60 to 80 beats per minute (bpm), typical of Baroque music, often produces a calming effect on our bodies. Music faster than 80 bpm can create an energizing effect. Much Western music—and this may be more than coincidence—is played at this tempo.

Composers of the Baroque era typically kept certain numbers and patterns in mind when they chose the beat, tempo, and harmony for their music. According to some reports, musicians in this period believed that particular sounds and rhythms could literally put human minds and bodies "in tune," producing healing, calming effects.

Some studies indicate that carefully selected music can enhance learning, memory, and concentration; reduce chronic pain by releasing endorphins; increase creativity; and alleviate stress.

Research also indicates that our heart rate synchronizes with music, speeding up or slowing down to match the tempo. Studies on the physiological effects of music also note that music affects respiratory rate, blood pressure, stomach contractions, hormone secretion, and the brain's electrical patterns.

This knowledge leads to many practical applications:

- Music played for people before, during, and after surgery diminishes anxiety and pain, reduces the need for medication, and speeds recovery.
- Dentists acknowledge the therapeutic effects of music when they allow people to listen to tapes or the radio during drilling and tooth extractions.

- It is increasingly common to play music for women during childbirth. The theory is that music reduces pain and may decrease the length of labor.
- Music therapy is a widely accepted field, used as part of programs to treat cancer, respiratory problems, stroke, arthritis, and diabetes. Music therapists have also reported success in working with autistic children.

Research in this area actively continues. There's even a new science—cymatics—devoted to studying the effects of different sounds and music on matter. In some of these studies, for example, researchers play sounds through solenoids (a type of magnet), and watch the patterns formed by metal filings near the solenoids. At certain sounds, filings assume geometrical shapes. It seems that even nonconscious matter can be patterned by the power of music.

Let's return to the subject of this book—exercise that helps you conduct yourself well! Music is standard fare in most aerobics classes. Instructors know that music lifts moods and helps regulate breathing. Moving to rhythm can help us stretch muscles smoothly and gradually increase endurance.

When we J'ARM, however, music is far more than a pleasant distraction that coaxes us into activity. Here music moves to the foreground, becoming a central part of the whole experience of exercise.

Though much of the research referred to in this chapter has been done with orchestral music, you do not have to limit yourself to Bach or any of the "classical" composers. Instead, you can choose the music that has the most positive effect on you. If you're looking for some ideas to start with, see the suggestions for music at the back of this book.

As a wellness advocate and physician, I strongly urge you to adopt a steady diet of pleasant music. Remember, pleasant music is a miracle drug without side effects. It puts a song in your heart, radiates joy on your face, reduces loneliness, recalls fond memories, fires up your brain, and boosts your energy level. Start today to develop a "sound library" of happiness-inducing selections. Use specially selected happy music to put more merriment in your life.

And when J'ARMING to popular songs, don't forget the lyrics. Even simple, popular songs like *"Oh, What a Beautiful Morning"* or *"Put on a Happy Face"* can encourage positive thoughts and raise our attitudes. To enhance the effects of music as you J'ARM, recite or sing the song lyrics in a bold voice. Go ahead and use some oxygen. Lift a ceiling or two.

J'ARMING to music is uplifting, both mentally and physically. When we listen to upbeat music and lyrics we often gain new energy. We feel better. A lot of problems can be forgotten during a beautiful song and a vigorous session of J'ARMING.

Tools of the trade

To become the great conductor of your "body orchestra" you need a baton. This can be imaginary, but it is preferable to be a bit more conventional and find a reasonable facsimile as you begin to J'ARM.

J'ARMERS have been very creative in using pens, pencils, knives, forks, spoons, brushes, and other implements. However, I prefer chopsticks. The chopstick seems to lend a special aura of talent and symbolizes the good health principles of healthy oriental cooking—high fiber and low fat.

If you want to become serious about "proper" baton

techniques, you can get a textbook on conducting from the library and study the fine points of this art. (You'll also find a few tips starting on page 46). As my friends will attest, however, my conducting technique has never been right, let alone proper. Almost any movement you come up with that appears close to the real thing is impressive—and healthful. And if your technique looks a little funny—what's the difference? It may even lead to laughter and raising the endorphins even more.

Again, remember that a real baton is nice, but not necessary. Other things you can J'ARM with include:
- Chopsticks
- Ball point pens
- Tongue blades
- Peacock feathers
- Spoons
- Back brushes in the shower
- Your hands
- Silk scarfs

When and where to J'ARM

Be creative looking for times and places you can J'ARM:
- In the shower
- While cooking. (Note: This is fun but it can get messy. Don't burn yourself!)
- While getting dressed
- First thing in the morning
- Just before lunch or dinner
- While in your car, sitting at a stoplight and listening to the radio. (Give the driver in the next car something to talk about when she gets home.)

■ In a private place at work for a few "feel good" moments of J'ARMING. Or better yet, J'ARM in a public place at work with some buddies.

In short, you can J'ARM just about any place at about any time. Even while lying still you can visualize yourself J'ARMING and enjoy some of the same benefits.

Basic J'ARM

J'ARMING is a unique exercise. First off, there are many things you do not need to J'ARM. You need no fancy clothing, no expensive shoes, no elaborate equipment, no special building, gym, or exercise facility. You need not learn any special technique, because you develop your own unique style. You can J'ARM anywhere, with or without clothing. (Careful with the latter option!)

You can J'ARM at any time, no appointments necessary. Nor do you need special lighting. In fact, you can J'ARM in the dark. You do not need a score board. No grades are given. Bad weather need not keep you from J'ARMING. Dogs need not nip at your heels, cars need not honk at or splash on you, and no salesperson will call to sell you a membership.

With apologies to Dr, Seuss, I offer this summary of the advantages of J'ARMING: You can do it in the dark, you can do it in the park, you can do it as a lark. You can do it in a chair, you can do it on a stair, you can do it with a flair, you can do it completely bare. You can do it here, you can do it there, you can do it—anywhere!

In Basic J'ARM 101 there are only two simple suggestions to follow. First, let go a little. Let yourself regress a bit. Get your arms moving, and approach this more as play than exercise.

Sometimes beginning J'ARMers feel they look silly. So look silly. What form of exercise doesn't look a little silly, anyway? Actually, it's the people who refuse to exercise who are truly being silly.

Second, choose some uplifting, invigorating music. Music with upbeat lyrics is ideal, because the positive message helps raise those "inner uppers," the endorphins. This is all you need to get started. It's really that simple. After several sessions of Basic J'ARMING, however, you may want to move on to the intermediate course.

Intermediate J'ARM

Now that you have mastered the basics, you can begin to exaggerate arm and body movement. Move your arms more vigorously, lift your arms higher, and widen the arc of your movements. With a real or imaginary baton, pretend it is ten inches from your hands, floating in the air. Reach for it with your arms and whole body. If you feel inclined, and if you've checked with your physician about doing so, you may want to add weights to your arms. Runners often use such weights, and you can generally find them in sports supply stores.

Next, devote some more attention to the music you're using. Again, each J'ARMer will develop his or her own favorite type of music. It may be classical, pop, jazz, country western, religious, or the Golden Oldies. Choose what feels right, whatever gives you an inner feeling of harmony. My only recommendation is that you J'ARM to a variety of music. That keeps the program fresh, as well as educational. (For more ideas, see "Suggestions for Music" on page 107.)

I'd also like you to experiment with singing as you J'ARM. Those who sing seem to experience some special "good vibrations." Vibrations of the voice may have special healing properties. Songs and chants are an important part of the ceremonies in almost all religions, and they're widely used to calm the body and center the mind. It's possible that the body "reads" these vibrations on a deep level. In some sacred traditions, singing is used to connect people with their natural surroundings, their fellow human beings, and their Creator.

At the every least, singing increases the aerobic effect of J'ARMING. When you sing, you use more oxygen. And you just might have more fun. Incidentally, don't worry if you're J'ARMING to orchestral or other instrumental music without words. Just sing along with the melody using simple syllables such as la, da, um, ho, he, ha, or make up your own lyrics. And if you don't feel like singing, whistle! Whatever you do, make noise. Be loud.

Two other quick suggestions are these. First, J'ARM with others whenever you can. The group spirit provides an extra incentive to maintain your program. Besides, exercising with others is often more fun than exercising alone, and you're bound to meet new people or deepen your existing friendships.

Also, J'ARM in front of a mirror—a full-length mirror if possible. There's a simple reason for this. Notice what happens when people standing in line or waiting for an elevator glance at themselves in a mirror. Often they'll make a few subtle movements to improve their appearance, such as standing or sitting up straighter. As you know, this posture preserves a healthful arch in your lower back. It also allows you to burn more calories than slumping or slouching. When you J'ARM in front of a mirror, you get instant and constant feedback on your stance. You can act on the feedback immediately.

So in review, Intermediate J'ARMING means including any of the following: exaggerated movements, singing, J'ARMING with others, or J'ARMING in front of a mirror. At this point, you're on your way to becoming a master J'ARMer. Work with these suggestions for a while. Then, stick around for Advanced J'ARM.

Advanced J'ARM

Unlike the conductors you see in the concert halls or on television, you will not be confined to a small step-up riser or platform when you conduct. Don't you feel sorry for conductors when the music almost shouts "move!" and they have to control themselves to maintain an artistic image? Imagine how the audience might react if a conductor would suddenly leap off the podium and dance or march across the stage!

Aren't you lucky that you have no such worries to contend with? And isn't it comforting to realize you don't have any talented artistic image to uphold? For me, having little or no talent can be a decided advantage. What I lack in musical talent I can make up for in spirited movement.

So if you can, move across the room when you J'ARM. You don't have to stay in a confined space. One of my fantasies is to J'ARM in a large dance hall or auditorium, with music from the sound system filling the whole place. As I J'ARM, I stroll, walk, dance, march, leap, jog, or even run from one end of the place to another. And there's nobody there to stop me or even notice what I'm doing.

You can do something like this at home. Feel free to move anywhere in your home, as long as you can still hear the music. J'ARM while moving from room to room or floor to floor. You'll just burn more calories as you do so.

Another simple but effective variation is to step up and step down on a step while J'ARMING. Or, walk up and down stairs as you J'ARM. Both methods increase the aerobic benefit and develop the upper leg and hip muscles.

Again, these are just optional suggestions. And if you do add such movements to your J'ARMING program, start slowly. Allow yourself to warm up.

I particularly like to J'ARM to a waltz and to dance with my partner in my living room. I make sure the candles are burning and the fireplace is blazing. J'ARMING with someone I care about really adds to the glow.

This works even if your partner is present only in your imagination. Friends relate how they have "called back" a lover and shared a J'ARMING evening. Jake, with a tear in his eye, tells me how he has J'ARMed and danced the night away with his departed loved one. He sets up the living room, showers, shaves, pours two glasses of wine, and takes one of her perfumed hankies to be used as a J'ARM baton. He starts playing an old Glenn Miller recording and begins to J'ARM. In his imagination he spiritually lives again in the presence of his departed wife. And she, this night, is the life of the party.

Here's another way to add movement. One popular variation is to J'ARM using a chair. Sit down in the chair, then rise from the seated position. Sit again. Then rise again. Keep repeating these movements, and keep your arms moving to the music the whole time. This is one exercise that helps keep people out of nursing homes. It builds muscle reserve in the upper leg and groin area—the muscles we use to sit down, stand up, and walk. Such up-down, up-down exercise keeps the "get up and go" muscles strong.

If you're feeling really adventuresome, then experiment with J'ARMING while sitting in a rocking chair or standing on a rocker board. You can find rocker boards at athletic stores or physical therapy supply stores. Balance or rock back and forth. Be cautious, however, with this one. And if you do use such a board, store it safely so others don't trip on it.

J'ARMING on a rocking surface, balancing on one leg, or with your eyes closed, helps you develop and maintain your sense of balance. This exercise makes use of your proprioceptors—the nerve endings that determine your orientation in space. Persons with good proprioceptors are usually better coordinated less likely to fall. If they do fall, they are better able to "steer" their fall and experience a soft landing.

My final recommendation is optional and more for those of you with an interest in music. If you like, J'ARM using the actual baton movements that professional conductors use. These movements vary according to the meter of the music—that is, the number of beats per measure. The simplest to conduct is music with two beats per measure. For example, marches such as "Stars and Stripes Forever" have two beats per measure. To conduct such music, a band director would make these movements:

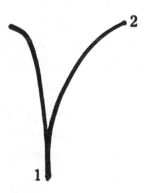

Another common meter is three beats per measure. This is also known as "waltz time." The Strauss Waltzes and popular songs like "Moon River" are written in waltz time. You can conduct this meter using the following movements:

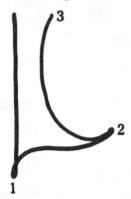

The other most common meter in Western music is four beats per measure. Most popular songs fall in this group. Here are the movements conductors usually use for this meter:

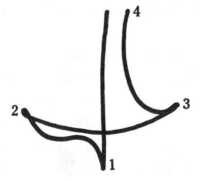

Special exercise challenges

As mentioned earlier, there is no incorrect way to J'ARM. As with any other form of exercise, however, some people encounter special challenges when they begin a J'ARMING program.

People with joint problems

Patients with lower extremity problems are urged to use the legs as much as possible. Some hip, knee, ankle, or foot conditions make that impossible. However, it's still wise to pursue the benefits of exercise. Non-weight-bearing exercise continues to be a must. Most of us do not have the luxury of swimming pools or stationary bicycles, but we can all stretch to help maintain muscle and joint tone. And we can J'ARM for cardiovascular fitness.

If you have neck and shoulder, arm, or hand pain, check with a physician or physical therapist before exercising. J'ARM movements are seldom harmful, but it's a good idea to ask and be sure.

I tell my patients that arms stiffen very rapidly when not used. If your shoulder has been weakened by disuse, start exercising slowly. Don't be afraid of mild pain, however. (That means pain at a level of one or two on a range of zero to ten, with zero being no and ten being a lot.) J'ARM for only three to five minutes at first to see how the shoulder and arm react at the time of the exercise, and on the next day.

People confined to a wheelchair or bed

Even if you are confined to a wheelchair or bed, you can still J'ARM. This form of exercise focuses on moving the arms—something you can do from a sitting or lying position. In hospital burn units, orthopedic wards, rehabilitation units, and nursing homes, people have used J'ARMING to condition both their minds and their bodies.

Stroke patients

It has been wonderful to see what J'ARMING can do for some stroke patients. Not only is the exercise beneficial, but the music has been shown to be a tool to help "reconnect" the left and the right sides of the brain. A happy J'ARM tune may just open a circuit and help speed stroke rehabilitation and recovery.

Back arching

In Chapter Two I mentioned the healthful effects of preserving an arch in your lower back, also know as the lumbar area. One person who came to see me referred to this area his "lumber area" because it was stiff as a board. You can pay attention to this position as you J'ARM.

To loosen the tight, rubber-band-like tissues in the back, we can start with gentle stretching exercises. Such exercises make it easier to experience the benefits of J'ARMING.

Tight tissues over the front of the body and front of the spinal column can slowly stretch out, helping us reposition the body into a more youthful, comfortable posture. Those who especially need arching exercises are people who have a low-back problems after long periods of sitting, while bending forward, or upon getting up in the morning. If such pain gets better with activities such as walking, then we have another clue that arching will be beneficial. (We tend to arch the back when we walk.)

Following are some steps you can take toward healthful back arching.

STEP ONE: Start by walking more—briskly for at least 20 minutes each day. If you tolerate walking well, then move on to Step Two.

STEP TWO: Standing with the buttocks against a stable object, such as a counter, table, or sturdy chair, bend backwards 10 times in 30 to 60 seconds. Arch the back until you feel a pull and a little discomfort. You may feel this stretch in both the back and front of the body.

If you think of discomfort on a pain scale of zero to ten, with zero being no pain and ten being a great deal, you should be feeling pain of between two and four. Mother Nature usually tells you the difference between healthy and unhealthy pain. If a sharp or shooting pain occurs in your back or legs, or if your back feels worse several hours after this movement, then stop the exercise and check with your physician. If this standing arch works well for you, move on to Step Three.

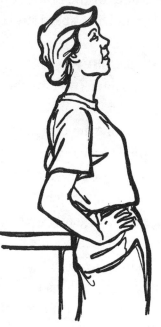

STEP THREE: Lie face down on the bed or floor with your hands in the "push-up" position. Keep your hip bone on or as near the floor as possible while you push up the upper body, arching the lower back.

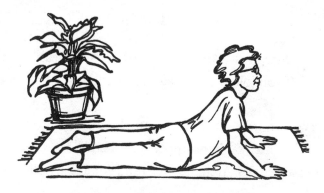

I tell my patients to do ten of these arch-ups in 30 to 60 seconds. The first seven are done rapidly, and the last three are done with the elbows held stiff and the low back/pelvis sagging as near the floor as possible. Hold the position for a count of five on each of the last three arches.

During the reconditioning-regenerating phase of back rehabilitation, this exercise should be done three times a day.

Another simple, easy way to do the low back arching stretch is to lie on the floor or bed on your stomach. Prop up your elbows and read a book or newspaper for several minutes.

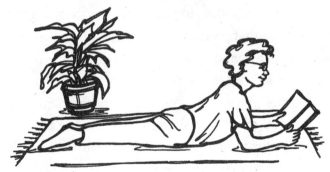

Posture habit retraining

J'ARMING is an excellent exercise for helping us get "back" into better posture. Have you noticed the posture of conductors and choir leaders? Many of them sit and stand erect, appearing flexible and vigorous. They often appear healthy and alive—much younger than their chronological age. It seems that their physiological (body) age and mental (mind) age have retained an enviable youthfulness.

As soon as the back starts to loosen, it's time to develop a new you—that is, a new posture habit. Your posture is largely the result of your sitting habits. For the most part, headaches, neck aches, backaches, and the "little old man" (LOM) and "little old lady" (LOL) looks are a consequence of poor sitting posture habits. The good news is that habits can be changed if we want to change them.

Think of a habit as a program running in our master computer—the brain. More importantly, remember that this program eventually becomes comfortable and runs on automatic. Before that can happen, however, we must send the proper reminder to our brains ("sit up straight, arch the low back"). That message has to be entered hundreds, perhaps thousands of times. Eventually, the automatic program can take over and run by itself. At that point, the program is on automatic and we sit up straight by habit. Usually converting to the new posture program takes about thirty days.

During the first week of posture habit retraining, we may need to "input" the "sit up straight, arch the low back" message to the computer 300 times a day. The second week, inputting that figure could drop 200 times a day, and the third week it may drop again to 100 times a day. Each day fewer messages will be required, and after thirty or forty days the automatic program kicks in. After that, only an occasional reminder is needed.

During this training program, you can use reminders to help you keep the arch. Just insert pillows, rolled up towels, or sweaters behind your lower back as you sit. Some chairs are specially designed to help you sit correctly.

One reminder I use is called the "lumbar roll." You can purchase this device in stores, or you can make it yourself. Simply roll up a bath towel and wrap tape around the towel to help maintain the shape. Then put this roll behind your lower back when you sit. Some patients lovingly refer to these homemade devices as their "couch potato." It's an apt name.

Another option is to make a lumbar roll that can be tied around your waist. Here's how:

Take a pair of womens' nylon stockings and slide a rolled up towel into the foot of one of the stockings. (I'll refer to this stocking as stocking #1.)

Then take the other stocking (call it stocking #2) and cut a tiny hole in the toe of it.

Next, take stocking #1 and slide the leg end inside the leg of stocking #2. Pull the leg of stocking #1 out through the toe hole of stocking #2.

Now pull stocking #2 all the way through stocking #1 until the rolled up towel ends up being in the foot of both stockings.

Finally, tie the leg ends of both stockings around your waist and knot them in the front.

Now you can wear this contraption around your waist. The rolled up towel will rest in the small of the back, serving both as a support and a reminder to sit up tall. You can even wear it over or under shirts and sweaters. Think of it as a healthful way to "tie one on."

Men who hesitate to wear nylon stockings to the office can ask a physician for a length of stockinette that is used as the first layer of casts. Place a rolled towel in the middle of the stockinette and tie the loose ends of the stockinette around your waist. This way the supportive towel can rest in the lumbar area of your back.

In short, help yourself get rid of the LOI/LOM hump—jutting chin, forward neck, rounded upper back and shoulders—by redeveloping and maintaining the inward arch of the lower back while sitting. When the low back arch (lumbar lordotic curve) is maintained, the rest of the body falls into position. You'll know you're in position when a side view of your body shows the "ear and the rear" to be in a straight line.

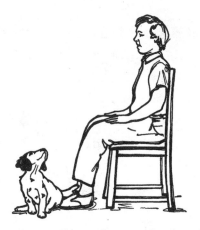

This healthy, sit-tall posture not only improves body mechanics—it can also help us lose weight. Sitting up straight is more work than sitting slouched. In an erect posture, we burn ten to fifteen additional calories an hour. Over a year, that's a potential loss of ten to fifteen pounds of fat. Posture habit retraining can help us look younger, stay or become slimmer, and at the same time takes away many aches and pains.

Tom (page 29) did the arching and stretching program outlined above and developed a much-improved posture. He told me that one day he picked up his baton, like a great orchestra leader, turned on some happy music, and started directing. At the same time, he found himself looking in the mirror and saying, "Thomas, young man, you're looking ... 'J'ARMING!'"

The Relaxing Stretch

The following technique can be used for a short period before or after J'ARMING to promote better muscle tone.

The relaxing stretch has been developed using the following basic principles:

- A muscle that is rarely used, along with its surrounding tissue, becomes tense, stiff, or spastic and tends to shorten. This limits motion.
- The shortened muscle, if stretched when irritated, may cause pain, but...
- If any muscle is used and then relaxed there is a "window of opportunity" during which the muscle becomes more cooperative. It releases some of its spasm and the tissues stretch (lengthen) with minimal or no pain.
- Once a muscle and its associated tissue is lengthened and then continually used, it tends to retain its new length and remain "loose."

The relaxing stretch is a comfortable way to gradually increase the length of a muscle and improve its flexibility. This technique will work with any tight muscle or group of muscles. (The following instructions illustrate the stretch using the hamstring and gluteal muscles in the left leg and hip.) Here's how:

STEP ONE: Lie on your back and bring the left knee gently to the chest until it meets slight resistance. This is the first site of tightness, also called the first barrier. There should be minimal or no pain at the barrier.

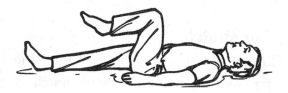

STEP TWO: After you reach this barrier, do not try to pull the knee any farther toward the chest. Instead of stretching the tight muscles, you are now going to tense and work the muscles.

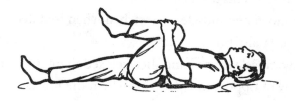

To do this, place both hands around the knee. Keep your hands stationary and push the knee out against the hands. You're not going anywhere—just tensing the hamstring and gluteal muscles that would normally straighten out the leg. (Note: You are now pushing in the opposite direction of the desired stretch. Make sure that the body stays stationary during this step.) Push the knee outward against your hands for about 5 seconds.

STEP THREE: Stop pushing and relax a few seconds.

STEP FOUR: Now pull your knee toward your chest. Because you've relaxed muscles that were just working, you can now stretch those muscles a little more. You'll probably be able to move your knee closer to your chest until you reach a new tightness barrier.

STEP FIVE: Repeat steps two to four.

The same technique works for any muscle or muscle and joint complex. I have found it especially useful for loosening a tight neck, shoulder, or leg. Each time you push against an unmoving counter force in the opposite direction from the desired stretch, you work the tight muscle. When you stop pushing, the muscle relaxes. During that brief period of relaxation, you can stretch the muscle.

People who first try this simple technique are usually amazed at how effective it is. Just remember to push against a fixed object in the opposite direction of the desired stretch. Relax, and then stretch again to a new tight barrier. Repeat this whole procedure three or four times. Using the Relaxing Stretch, you can really become a "loose" man or woman.

Responding to pain

Earlier I mentioned the role of endorphins in relieving pain. There's more to be said, however, about the whole subject of pain and exercise. Many of us have negative feelings about exercise—usually because we think of it as that awful four-letter word work. The old saying "no pain, no gain" has scared us into believing we must go through suffering and self-flagellation before we can reap the benefits of exercise.

Yes, some minor pain may be associated with exercise. But it is usually temporary. A few minor aches and pains are to be expected the day after we start to reuse some deconditioned muscles. If we keep the pos"I"tive image of our goal in mind, we'll learn to see this training pain as a little hurtful, but not harmful.

Often the people who come to see me, particularly the VPS (vintage people) complain of a great deal of motion restriction and pain when certain movements are pushed to the limit. Peggy said, "We are told to stretch, but often it's too painful. I stop, because I question whether I'm hurting myself."

I said, "Peggy, when it comes to muscular and skeletal pain (biomechanical pain), the question should not be, am I hurting myself, but rather, am I harming myself?"

Maybe you've been told "if it hurts, don't use it." This common, often misguided advice has been oversold. The wise exerciser understands there are two kinds of mechanical, or movement, pain. Good pains are those that hurt only temporarily and get better with time. However, some harmful pains last much longer and can get progressively worse, becoming detrimental to general health. These bad pains have the potential to shorten life.

Good (hurtful) pain

Pains that occur at the end of movement and have a "stretch" quality I usually consider as "good" pains. Those stretch pains that convey a message from Mother Nature that says, "yes, your body needs that," are the kind that we can continue. This is pain that we can work through. Indeed, such pain may be necessary in exercising and conditioning to improve overall health.

John was concerned with the pains he was getting in his knees with walking and in his shoulders and arms with J'ARMING He asked, "How hard should I push myself? Am I hurting myself?"

"Yes, John, you are hurting yourself, but you are not harming yourself," I replied. "In all likelihood we can enhance your general cardiovascular conditioning and lessen your everyday aches and pains if we proceed with a program in which you control your degree of acceptable discomfort."

Bad (harmful) pain

Bad or harmful pains are those that can herald or result in a serious life-threatening or life-shortening event. For example, a pain in the chest or shoulder that comes on during or after exercise and cannot be made better or worse by body movement could be heart-related. People who experience such pain need to see a physician.

Any chronic or low grade pain that is not clearly related to or aggravated by movement could be a harmful pain. And pain that arises acutely for no apparent reason can be serious whether it is related to movement or not.

Severe pain in a joint that makes you slow down or stop an activity is also harmful pain. This is not so much because such pain signals damage in the joint, but because the pain too often prompts the person to "slow down" which]can lead to a general deconditioning of the essential heart, lungs, and brain.

People with "bad knees" often ask me if they should still keep walking, even with their pain. I tell them to avoid as much jarring of the joint as possible, walk with a light step, and wear shoes with good shock absorbers. But, yes, for the benefit of general health of their muscles, heart, lungs, (as well as mental health and weight control) they should exercise. This is true even though they have pain. Knee joints are replaceable; the heart is not. I have never seen someone die of a knee attack.

"Severe pain" is a relative, individual, subjective interpretation of a body sensation. Everyone has his or her own pain "threshold," and what is severe to one person may be only annoying to another. I have worked with patients who have had pain that would have agonized someone else, and yet not complain. Others scream when they put on aftershave lotion or wince when their hair is touched.

All bodies are different, and so are the ways they experience pain. That's why it is so important to read your body's signals and determine your individual tolerance. Again, to do this, develop your own "Scale of Pain" with a range of zero to ten. Zero is no pain and ten is screaming, hair-pulling pain. Each of us needs to try to keep the quantity of pain to level three or less. Anything above that could well be harmful pain.

Seeing the difference between good and bad pain

We also needed to look at the quality of the pain. Is it sharp-stabbing or dull-aching? Is it constant or intermittent? Are there other signs of distress or illness? Is it getting progressively worse or better? What position makes the pain better or worse? Is it worse during activity or at rest? Does the pain get worse or better with stretching? Does cold, heat, or the weather affect it? Are any medications helpful? In short, what makes the pain better or worse?

Answering these questions with your physician will almost always guide you to a useful assessment of your pain. If your physician or physical therapist helps you understand that your pain is hurtful and not harmful, then keep going. Push yourself for the sake of your health. This is much like riding a bicycle. We have to keep pedaling, even when pain makes it harder to go up hill. But we still learn to balance pain with the benefits of conditioning—or over we go.

Any pain could be bad. But for the most part, an intermittent pain that is related to body movement and can be improved with body movement I consider to be a hurtful (good) and not a harmful (bad) pain. Pain that gets better with activity I usually consider merely a hurtful pain.

Many aches and pains experienced by J'ARMERS and other active people are related to a tightness or spasm in a muscle or muscle group. These aches and pains often mysteriously disappear "overnight" when we sleep like a baby. The body mobilization technique Fold and Hold, described in my book *Muscle Pain Relief in 90 Seconds* (Chronimed Publishing), demonstrates how many of these common, irritating aches and pains can be eliminated with simple, natural, safe, and nonhurtful body positioning.

Ways to supplement your J'ARMing program

Other exercises that use the arms can offer benefits similar to J'ARMING. Try any of the following activities as ways to add variety to your J'ARMING program:

- Play tennis
- Swim
- Jump rope
- Bowl
- Do carpentry
- Paint houses
- Wash windows

- ■ Juggle
- ■ Play horseshoes
- ■ Play volleyball, basketball, baseball, bocce ball, handball, lacrosse, squash, or racquetball
- ■ Dance
- ■ Do handstands
- ■ Do Tai Chi
- ■ Work out with weights or pulleys
- ■ Do pull-ups
- ■ Go cross-country skiing
- ■ Wash and wax your car
- ■ Trim hedges
- ■ Play the violin or piano

In addition, you can do some short exercises designed specifically for the arms. These include arm circles, punching air, riding the bicycle, and the Codman exercises.

Note: Watch for these signs while doing any exercises that involve shoulder movement: numbness in your hands, a feeling of weakness in your arms, or lightheadedness. A condition called subclavian steal, caused by blockages in the arteries going to the arms, can cause troublesome drainage of blood going to the head. This can lead to lightheadedness and, in rare cases, even a stroke. If you feel any of these symptoms, stop the exercise immediately. Get medical attention.

ARM CIRCLES: Stand with your arms out to your sides. Make little circles with your full arms. Gradually make the circles smaller and smaller. Do the circles faster as you make them smaller.

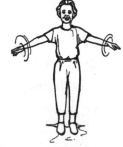

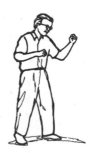

PUNCHING AIR: Like arm circles, this exercise is a great de-stresser. Pretend that you are a boxer and throw left and right punches into the air. Punch fast and slow, high and low.

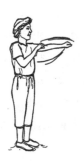

RIDING THE BICYCLE: Move your arms as if they were legs pedaling a bicycle.

THE CODMAN EXERCISES: If you find it difficult to move your shoulders, then consider doing the Codman exercises. Bend forward and let your arms hang like a pendulum. Then swing your arms in different directions—backward, forward, side-to-side, or in circles.

And always—the laughter prescription

As another way to round out their J'ARMING program, I often give my patients a laughter prescription. I actually write out a prescription with words to this effect: "Stand in front of the mirror and belly laugh for fifteen seconds, three times each day."

What we're talking about here is no ordinary laugh. I mean an all-out, bellowing, no-holds-barred belly laugh. Not just a little twitter but a belly-holding, gut-busting, gas-passing guffaw.

Often people say, "Oh, I really can't do it. My family is going to laugh at me." They're probably right. Their families will laugh at them. But soon their families will start laughing with them, because there is nothing more contagious than this prime endorphin-raising activity.

Try it right now before reading any further. Just put your book down for a minute and stand right where you are. Now for fifteen seconds, laugh as hard as you can. Really let yourself go. Better yet, do this with friends and family members. Go ahead and raise a roof, and feel the difference.

Hard to stop, isn't it? Once you try the laughter prescription, your body will ask you for more. Soon you'll find yourself making time for gut-busting belly laughs at least once a day. After we laugh, our muscles relax. Heartbeat and blood pressure decrease, signs of reduced stress. This parallels with what happens to the body after exercise. Indeed, laughter is a kind of internal jogging.

Occasionally someone says to me, "Look, I'm not going to take this belly laughing prescription. I just don't really quite grab onto that." "Fine," I reply. "Here is something else you can try. Just put a smile on your face. Do it right now. Feels good, doesn't it?" I believe you can almost feel those endorphins raising when you smile. Smiles, like laughs, are contagious, prompting the saying "Grin and share it."

The day goes the way the corners of the mouth go. We can, by putting a smile on our face, get better "smileage" out of life. It's more important what you wear from ear to ear than what you wear from head to toe. I sum it up by saying that smiling is a free way to increase your "face value"—an investment that pays high dividends. We already know that when you wrap a gift in high-quality wrapping paper or put an attractive frame on a picture, then people tend to perceive the package or picture as being more valuable. This is also the case when people put smiles on their faces.

I know people who get up in the morning, go to the window, look out to check the weather and groan, "Good God—morning." Other people look out and say the same three words in a different way: "Good morning, God." The second group of people usually begin the day with a smile on their faces. They make their own weather. This self-made weather becomes the "climate" of their existence and a significant factor in the emotional "environment" not only in their lives but in the lives of those about them. Our actions and feelings are contagious. Each day we can ask ourselves often, "What will I spread today?"

I used to believe that the posture of the body and the expression on the face resulted from a the way a person felt. In other words, you feel happy, then you smile. But now I'm learning that I had it backwards. New studies are showing that feelings can follow the "prompting" of a body position. If you smile, you can feel better. People have been asked by researchers to frown and then write down the first thought that comes into their heads. For most people, that thought is a neutral or negative thought. But ask them to smile and that first thought changes to a positive, affirming, optimistic thought.

Why go into such detail on the laughter prescription and the virtues of smiling? Because I consider them essential to J'ARM-ING. When you J'ARM, smile and laugh. Both actions enhance the physical and emotional benefits of the exercise. Like many others, you may naturally find yourself laughing when you J'ARM. In that case, just keep up the good work. You've graduated from our J'ARM university and won a lifetime scholarship to good health.

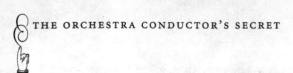

J'ARMing and the New Science of Health

A cheerful heart is a good medicine,
but a downcast spirit dries up the bones.
—Proverbs 17:22

WITH OVER FORTY YEARS IN MEDICINE, I'VE SEEN SOME PEOPLE give up and let their health progressively deteriorate. I've also seen many more take their illness or pain and turn it around. The question is: Why? Why can some people gain control, take charge of their health, and emerge victorious? Is there, as in many aspects of life, a "winner's edge," a decisive spurt of effort that promotes lasting health? Do we each have a "physician within," as some claim, an internal source of healing that we can invoke? That you can "conduct" on?

My answer is yes. There's nothing strange, mystical, or "new age" about this idea (though the word "miraculous" seems appropriate at times). We are merely discovering that the mind and emotions play a decisive role in physical health. In fact, the whole new area of research called *psychoneuroimmunology* (PNI) has evolved to study this phenomenon closely. Again, don't let that long, complicated name intimidate you. This field is really about things we experience every day, and you don't have to be a scientist to take advantage of its findings.

Psychoneuroimmunology is the area that Bernie Siegel, author of *Love, Medicine, and Miracles*, explored as he witnessed people who survived cancer. It's also the territory mapped by Norman Cousins, an author who used laughter and positive emotions to help recover from a life-threatening collagen illness. Interest in the body-mind connection has moved well into mainstream medicine, and solid research on this connection is now emerging.

I do not claim that everyone can reverse cancer, heart disease, multiple sclerosis or other diseases solely by changing their attitudes and emotions. Yet I will say that our minds and hearts can enter fully into the healing process—far more so than we used to think.

What are the details of that process? We don't have all the answers, but we can point in some promising directions. Among them are the placebo effect, choosing positive attitudes, and the power of imaging. Each of these can be applied to your J'ARM-ING program.

The placebo effect

My experience of the placebo effect dates back to my childhood in Austin, Minnesota. Austin is a small town in rural, southern Minnesota. I didn't realize it then, but a meaningful part of my medical education began in this friendly environment, the roots of my rich Scandinavian heritage.

I remember hearing certain phrases over and over again

when I was a boy: "It's all in the head." "Imagine that." "Isn't that touching?" At the time I did not understand that they contained profound medical wisdom.

The first time I remember hearing "it's all in the head" was in the heated discussion that surrounded Mrs. Becker's "miracle" cure. Mrs. Becker lived two houses down the road from us. She had been on crutches all the time that I had known her. A frenzied search for help had taken her from physician to physician, but each search failed to restore her health.

At last she decided to see the "touch doctor" who made a weekly visit to Rose Creek, a town about ten miles south of Austin. One Thursday afternoon, after a visit to the touch doctor, Mrs. Becker returned without her crutches. She had left them in in Rose Creek. I never saw her on crutches again.

I was ten years old when this happened, a time I mark as the beginning of my medical education. And I can still hear my Aunt Vera talking about Mrs. Becker. Every family must have an Aunt Vera. My own is someone whose wonderful laugh resounds in my mind even though she's been gone many years. Aunt Vera would roll her eyes, shake her head a bit, and laugh. "Ha, ha, ha, ha. Mrs. Becker—she went off to see the touch doctor. Isn't that touching? Left her crutches there in Rose Creek. Obviously whatever she had all these years was all in the head. Imagine that."

About the same time, one of my cousins graduated from college and went to Europe. He brought back photographs of all the places he'd visited. The ones I remember most vividly were pictures of Lourdes, a Roman Catholic shrine in southwest France. These pictures showed much cast-off paraphernalia of ill health—thousands of crutches, braces, canes, and wheelchairs. To an impressionable lad of ten, this was truly remarkable.

In 1858, legend has it, the Virgin Mary appeared at Lourdes to a fourteen-year old peasant girl, now known as St. Bernadette. Each year three million people visit Lourdes, many of them on crutches, braces, or wheelchairs and hoping for a miracle like the one that happened to St. Bernadette. Many of these people report "cures" after their visit to the holy site.

You can guess the prevailing opinion of my family about those pictures. They simply echoed Aunt Vera: "Those people who get cured that way—well, whatever they had was (ha, ha) all in the head. Imagine that."

Years later, when I was in medical school, I took part in testing new experimental pain medications. It was standard procedure in these studies to give one group of patients a placebo, a simple sugar pill that had no medicinal properties whatever. These patients, however, thought they were getting a powerful new pain medication. Another group of patients took a "real" new pain medication. Later we compared results from people taking the actual medication with results from those who'd taken the placebo.

To our surprise, the sugar pill effectively relieved pain about 40 percent of the time. By contrast, the actual pain medication was about 75 percent effective. Keeping with standard research practice, we threw out the results from the placebo. The placebo effect was a contaminant, we thought, caused by "tricks of the mind." Our reaction was merely a sophisticated version of Aunt Vera's: Obviously, anyone who experienced pain relief with a placebo had a condition that was "all in the head." Imagine that.

Looking back on this, I question why we didn't get excited about the apparent benefit of the placebo. It's obvious to me now that in medicine we need more scientific data on why the placebo works. Fortunately recent studies of the endorphins are shedding much light on this area.

After my training in general surgery at the Mayo Clinic, I went to Ethiopia as a member of the Peace Corps. To say that we were stretched thin is an understatement. There were twenty million people in Ethiopia, and I was one of nineteen physicians there at the time.

We would go on medical safaris to many of the remote Ethiopian villages to give small pox vaccinations and other immunizations to the children. Villagers would often ask us to see and care for some of their leaders. Often we had little more than aspirin, vitamin tablets, and some malaria pills.

At one of these villages a group appeared with their chief, who was complaining of weakness and pains. These people demanded more than just a pill for the chief: "Doesn't the American doctor have a shot?" They were becoming quite insistent. Indeed, I was concerned and somewhat frightened by their demands.

Fortunately that day in my doctor's "bag of tricks" I did have a syringe with a relatively large needle and a vial of 50% glucose (sugar) water. I simply drew two cubic centimeters of the sugar water into my syringe and administered a shots in the buttocks of one of the leaders. Sugar water has a special sting, so he felt the "power" of the medicine.

When I returned several months later, I was greeted with a cry: "Where's the American doctor? He was here and gave me that magic shot and today I feel so much better!" Of course, I knew, along with the other Peace Corps volunteers, that it was "all in the head." Unfortunately, Vera wasn't there to add, "Ha, ha, ha—imagine that."

The next step in my career was a position with the Indian

Health Service in Gallup, New Mexico. I was a surgeon working with the Hopi, the Navajo, and the Zuni Indians. It was common on the night before a Navajo went for surgery to find their medicine men in our ward, dressed in beads, feathers, and full healing regalia. These practitioners of the Navajo healing ceremony danced around the bed of the Navaho patients, singing sacred chants. And almost always, the Navaho patients who received such treatment recovered more quickly and with fewer complications than patients who did not get visits from the "dancing healers."

Years later I worked in the Biomechanic Clinic of a large medical clinic in Minneapolis. I saw many people with chronic aches and pains. Some of them, after living with a pain in their back or joints for three or four months, were referred to me. They called my receptionist and said, "I can't take it any more. I have to get in to Dr. Anderson and see what this pain is all about." Sometimes my receptionist said, "I'm very sorry but the earliest I can get you in is three weeks from today." I regretted such delays, and so did the people who called me. But they usually waited, and finally I did get to see them.

When the date of the office visit finally arrived, I greeted these people and asked them to tell me about the pain they had been living with. "Well, here we are. Now, what's the problem?"

At this point the patient often appeared a little nervous, perhaps a little bewildered. "I hate to say it, but that pain I called about—you know, the one I've had for three weeks? Well, I'm finally here to see you and... well... this is a good day. I feel much better. You know Doc, people always feel better the day they go see the doctor. Maybe it's all in the head."

As I listened to those words, I stood there at an impressive clinic in my official-looking white coat and other medical regalia

of the modern healer. I was seeing people who have been scheduled by my official-sounding receptionist. Close to my office was
a medical laboratory and rooms full of high-tech equipment—
part of the armamentarium of modern medicine. All this, even
though I hadn't touched the person in front of me yet, and she
was already feeling better.

I'm a little bewildered by all this—perhaps even a little
scared, because the touch doctor who came through Rose Creek
when I was ten years old was eventually run out of town. And
now, over fifty years after seeing that healing "miracle" in Rose
Creek, I wonder: Did Mrs. Becker have an illness that was "in the
head" or did she have a cure that was "in the head"?

Confronted with such questions, I often ask, Why? Why do
people experience relief from shots of sugar water, medicine men,
and "dummy" sugar pills? Why do they feel better after merely
making a medical appointment or entering a physician's office?

Currently we're getting some answers. And many of those
answers center on the "placebo effect"—the role that belief plays
in the relief of symptoms and the cure of disease. (The word
placebo comes from the Latin word, meaning "I shall please.")
The placebo effect says, in effect, that our hopes, expectations,
faith, and confidence in the "healer" may often be as important
as the medication or treatment we receive.

In their book *Healthy Pleasures*, brain researcher Robert
Ornstein and physician David Sobel review research on the
placebo effect. Their conclusion: Placebos are potent medicines
that have relieved headaches, coughs, toothaches, postoperative
pain, angina, asthma, warts, and other conditions. "It appears,"
they write, "that no symptom or system is immune to the
placebo effect."

Ornstein and Sobel cite one study of a woman suffering from severe nausea and vomiting. After trying several conventional treatments, which failed, her physicians said they were giving her a "new and extremely powerful wonder drug." This drug, they said, was certain to relieve her nausea. Twenty minutes after taking this drug, the woman's nausea disappeared.

What was the wonder drug? Syrup of ipecac, a medicine long used to induce vomiting. Here the placebo effect was powerful enough to reverse the normal effect of the medication.

It's no longer surprising to me when I read studies concluding that a 35 to 45 percent reduction of pain comes from the placebo effect alone. We know that people can get excellent results from ingesting a simple sugar or starch pill. Today, placebos are no longer dismissed as "quack remedies." Medical researchers are beginning to acknowledge their medicinal power, even though we don't understand how they work. It could be that placebos stimulate the brain, endocrine system, and adrenal glands to act in ways that heal the body.

Also, placebos may alleviate pain by triggering the release of endorphins. Evidence for this possibility comes from a study of people who underwent dental surgery to extract wisdom teeth. They received an intravenous injection of what they were told was a "very powerful" pain medication. In reality, that medication was a placebo. Forty percent of these people reported significant relief of pain. In addition, blood analysis confirmed that they experienced a rise in endorphins.

Next, the same group was given Nalaxone, a drug that blocks morphines and morphine-like chemicals such as endorphins. These people immediately reported an increase in pain, supporting the idea that endorphins were responsible for the pain relief.

"Whatever the precise pathways through mind and body," writes Norman Cousins in *Anatomy of an Illness,* "enough evidence already exists to indicate that placebos can be as potent as—and sometimes more potent than—the active drugs they replace."

More evidence for the power of belief in healing comes from the *nocebo effect,* the polar opposite of the placebo effect. If positive expectations can affect the course of therapy, so can negative expectations. In fact, negative beliefs may induce illness even when tests give no evidence of "real disease" in the body.

Larry Dossey, a physician with the Dallas Diagnostic Association, provides an example of the *nocebo effect* in his book *Space, Time and Medicine.* A man named Jim entered the hospital with an admitting diagnosis of cancer. He had lost fifty pounds in six months. Emaciated and weak, Jim wore what Dossey calls the "look of death." This was tragic enough. Yet even more distressing to Jim's physicians was another fact: Two weeks of the usual diagnostic tests showed no sign of cancer. All results were normal. Jim was dying, and his physicians had no idea why.

Eventually Jim confessed that he knew the reason for his condition. "Doctor," he said, "I've been hexed." According to Jim, an enemy had hired a shaman to steal a lock of Jim's hair and put a curse on it. According to the shaman, this meant Jim was doomed to die, and Jim believed so, too. The day he found out about the hex, Jim stopped eating. He'd come to the hospital to die.

Jim's physician, aware that every conventional medical treatment had failed, tried the only option he could think of: a midnight ceremony to "de-hex" Jim. During this ceremony, the physician cut another lock of Jim's hair and burned it. While this took place, the physician said, "As the fire burns your hair, the hex in your body is destroyed. But if you reveal this ceremony to any-one, the hex will return immediately, stronger than before!"

Jim took part in the ceremony with a combination of terror and respect. More importantly, he fully accepted the power of the de-hexing ceremony. He awoke the next morning and ordered a triple serving of breakfast and double servings of each following meal. After several days, Jim left the hospital as a well man, leaving behind a stack of normal test results.

Choosing positive attitudes

The placebo effect brings to mind another aspect of positive belief. It's been shown that beneficial body physiology—such as endorphins—can be "faked" up. For instance, forcing a smile or a laugh, according to many of the scientists working in this field, will fool the endorphins and other beneficial body chemicals into increasing. That's certainly a great reason for laughing more, even if the situation isn't necessarily that funny. Consciously being more optimistic and looking for the humor-ous side of every day events can give us that "inner high."

Be forewarned that if you talk about faking good feelings, you might be accused of being a Pollyanna, of seeing the world through rose-colored glasses, or being an incurable optimist. Even worse, a friend may say you're "in denial."

I know what it feel likes to be on the receiving end of this crit-icism. My reply is that Pollyanna got a bad rap. Consider this: All of us live by illusions. None of us really sees the world as it is. Instead, we see the world as we are.

There's a physiological reason for this. One of the main jobs of the human brain is to filter out a vast array of sense impres-sions. Those perceptions are coming at us at the rate of hundreds per second. Suppose you could be conscious of every thought, sight, sound, smell, taste, and body sensation you experienced. Talk about being burned out—you'd be on sensory overload!

Mercifully, our brains filter out most sense impressions so we can concentrate on what matters most. Think of the brain as a file clerk who can move faster than the speed of light. This clerk sorts our perceptions into piles marked "attend to this first," "act on this later," and, "ignore." But what determines which sense impressions go into the "attend to this first" pile? There are many factors, but our attitudes and general view of the world play a central role.

Take the student who has a passionate conviction that his career options are limited. What news stories is he more apt to notice? Chances are they'll be the latest unemployment figures, plant closings, and layoffs. In short, he takes in data that confirms his existing view of the world. This, in turn, discourages him from putting effort into career planning and job hunting.

Now take another student with roughly the same abilities and interests. Her general outlook is different, however. She believes her career options are virtually limitless, provided she plans carefully and cultivates her favorite skills. When she opens the morning paper, she's more likely to focus on stories that confirm her view: tips for successful interviewing and resumes, articles on interesting places to work.

Which person is right about the possibilities of personal success? It's impossible to prove either person right or wrong in any final sense. Perhaps both of their views are illusory to some degree. Yet which person is more likely to experience career satisfaction?

I'd place my bets with the optimistic woman. Many professionals in career planning hold that successful job hunting is primarily a function of choice, commitment, and action. The person with the optimistic outlook is more likely to display these qualities. Perhaps she is living by an illusion, but her illusions serve her well.

Many of the crucial issues of life present us with such options. The philosopher William James once said that he could not conclusively prove whether human beings have free will. Yet he decided to act on the idea that he had free will, because this view led to a more satisfying life. He, too, chose the "illusion" that served him best.

I go into this point in some detail because of the role that optimism and favorable attitudes play in raising endorphins and creating good health. We're learning more about this all the time. For example, psychologist Suzanne Kobasa and her colleagues at the University of Chicago studied executives at at&t when that company was undergoing corporate reorganization. This was a time of great stress for most at&t managers. Yet some executives remained generally healthy, while others succumbed to a variety of illnesses.

Kobasa concluded that the more healthy executives had a set of attitudes focused on three qualities. First, they had strong commitment to work and family. Second, they felt they were still in control of the overall quality of their lives. They lived by the saying, "If it is to be, it is up to me." And finally, they viewed change as a challenge rather than a threat. In short, these people lived by a set of optimistic assumptions—attitudes that registered in their bodies as well as their minds.

Before leaving this topic of positive attitudes and health, I want to make one more point. I'm excited by the groundswell of interest in the role of visualization, laughter, affirmations, prayer, and positive emotions in helping people overcome life-threatening diseases. At the same time, we cannot expect to smile automatically or laugh ourselves to perfect health. It's regrettably easy for people to inflict feelings of failure on themselves if they're unable to bring about miracle cures through these methods.

Self-blame can enter here. People who suffer certain illnesses such as cancer or repeated infections might blame themselves for harboring negative attitudes and failing to relate to people. They can get the idea that malignant tumors are something they wished or secretly willed upon themselves through flawed lifestyles. True, lifestyle is a crucial component of health. Yet we must emphasize that any illness has many facets and many causes. Rarely is one aspect of our lifestyle the sole cause of a disease. Obviously, factors such as sanitation, air and water quality, accidents, genetics, and many more can play a significant role outside of our individual control.

To say that the mind and emotions contribute significantly to physical health is not to say they are the only factors involved. Rather, many factors are at work in developing any state of health: exercise, nutrition, alcohol abuse, caffeine abuse, smoking, shift work, poor sleep, negative attitudes, financial problems, accidents, genetics, feeling out of control or unconnected to people. Any one of these many factors piled on top of other existing factors may be only the proverbial "straw that broke the camel's back" to cause disease.

I find it most constructive to concentrate on what people can do in the present to improve their health, along with the meaning and quality of their lives. This approach is far more effective than speculating on the ways they might have "created" an illness.

The power of imaging

"Rent or buy one of our costumes. Put it on… and become someone else!"

Several years ago, I saw this headline on a billboard outside a costume store in Tucson shortly before Halloween. How true, I thought. If only I could persuade more of my patients to change their "mental costume," they could feel so much better. My practice and those of my colleagues could be altered significantly if only patients would learn to use their pos"I"tive "ME"ntal "I"mages. If only they would bel"I"eve in their own inner powers of self healing. If only they could accept that self-talk and even acting can be keys to better health.

"The me I see is the me I'll be!" has been the theme of many motivational books and programs. The value of positive imaging is well accepted and practiced in school, business, and athletics. Yet our image of our future health is too often negative.

Judy, age fifty-two, is a very competent, hard-driving office manager. Like many people, she had a consuming fear that her nagging back pain was a serious, deteriorating problem that would get progressively worse. Judy saw herself becoming a LOL (little old lady), confined to a wheelchair. This image depressed her. And because she felt depressed, she assumed the body language of depression: slumped shoulders, trunk slouching forward. This, in turn, increased her odds of becoming precisely what she feared. I knew the only way we could turn this cycle around was to break the negative fearful image.

Many of Judy's friends would say she felt depressed, so she looked depressed. But could it really be the other way around? Judy looked depressed, so she felt depressed. Her negative body language made it easier for her to think negative thoughts and feel negative emotions. Actors and actresses understand that the body "makes the mind." They know that "putting on" the body "costume" of a desired emotion can create that emotion in the mind.

I asked Judy to think of me as her acting coach. She was now in acting school, and we were going to prepare her for several different parts. For each of the parts, I would ask her to assume an exaggerated body posture that would depict the character.

First I asked Judy to play a sad, despondent young woman. For this role, Judy sat slouched forward, head bent down, forehead wrinkled, corners of the mouth turned down, shoulders rolled forward, with shallow, short, inward breathing. In this position her body was folding inward on itself. Even Judy's breathing seemed to turn inward in short, choppy wheezes. Her thoughts, too, started to be turned inward. And because her body was in the sad position or "costume," her thoughts and speech patterns naturally developed along those negative lines.

I asked Judy what she was feeling and thinking. She almost broke into tears. How alone she felt, how out of touch, how apart from the world she felt. She thought of unpleasant relationships and personal failures in her life. Masterfully she assumed the role of a worried, dejected, defeated person.

Next I assigned Judy a new role—that of a bubbly, vigorous, successful woman of fifty-five who has just won the lottery and rekindled a romance with her high school sweetheart.

Judy immediately sat up straight, her shoulders back, her head and neck held proudly. Judy's ear and rear were in the perfect vertical alignment of erect posture. There was a twinkle in her eyes. A grin came to her face, and she even found herself laughing. Her hands and arms were held out. Her body appeared open, receptive, blossoming. Her breathing deepened and projected outward. She was filled with spark, fire, life.

"Oh, Judy. You're the perfect person for this part," I said. "What are you feeling? What are you thinking?"

You guessed it. She was experiencing wonderful feelings of happiness and good health—thoughts of love, optimism, and hope. By repositioning her body, Judy had put on the "body costume" of happiness and created a new body-image. That image was conveyed to her brain, which responded with positive thoughts, and the body, with positive physiological chemicals.

Test this for yourself. Have you ever stood in front of the mirror, feeling glum and not liking what you see and the way you feel? The next time you do, smile at yourself. Then stand straighter, vertically aligning your ear and your rear. Next, monitor your thoughts and feelings. See how difficult it is to sustain negative attitudes when you assume this new body stance.

Chances are that this simple exercise will help you see a new you. Mirrors are effective tools, and many studies point to improved productivity and energy levels in people who can "talk themselves up" by glancing in the mirror. I urge you to keep a mirror near the places where you dress, work, and relax. Use it as a reminder to put on the costume of happiness. After all, the best piece of costume jewelry is a big smile.

You can also hold this self-image in your mind, even when you're away from the mirror. When you're feeling depressed or lazy, visualizing yourself in the costume of happiness can dilute those negative feelings and clear a path for optimism and joy.

How these discoveries can help you J'ARM

Why all this emphasis on placebos, positive attitudes, and self-image in a book about J'ARMING? Because each of these techniques points to a way to enhance your J'ARMING program.

In some ways, exercise works much like the placebo effect: For one, it stimulates endorphin production. Exercise also alters moods for the better. Counselors know that people can often break a bout of depression merely by taking a walk or jogging through a park. I suggest you consciously use the placebo effect to your advantage. Tell yourself that J'ARMING is going to make a real difference in your health and the quality of your life. Affirm the effectiveness of this form of exercise, even if the affirmation feels forced at first. Soon your mind and body will overcome their initial resistance to change. If you don't feel it—well, fake it. If you still don't feel it, then fake it again... and again ... and again. Live out the old saying: Fake it until you make it. That's how habits are made.

Also use positive images. Create a detailed mental picture of the person you want to be. See yourself performing daily tasks with vigor and enthusiasm. Picture yourself at your ideal weight, standing erect, smiling, and laughing with the people you love. When creating this image, be as concrete as possible. Note what you will look like, what you will see, how you will stand, and how you will talk.

One of the most effective ways of getting the endorphin prescription from our internal pharmacy is to J'ARM. J'ARMING can do even more than give us good exercise. It can help us think happy, positive thoughts. It can get us laughing. It can help connect us with great music and with fellow J'ARMERS. It can help us recall pleasant memories and transform our self-image. If we believe in the benefits of J'ARMING, we will increase our rewards.

You can create your own prescription for feeling good. Put on the conductor's "costume" and J'ARM.

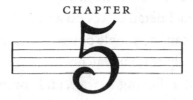

CHAPTER

How to Extend the Benefits of J'ARMing—
Becoming a C Personality

Think of persons as adventures.
—Lawrence Durrell

IN 1974 A BOOK APPEARED THAT CHANGED THE WAY AMERICANS talked about health. The title of that book was *Type A Behavior and Your Heart.* In this groundbreaking work, Meyer Friedman and Ray Rosenman described the close relationship between certain behaviors and the risk of coronary heart disease.

Friedman sums up the book's message with a single sentence: "Coronary heart disease cannot be due simply to what a person ingest or inhales; what he thinks and feels must also play a part."

What are the thoughts, feelings, and actions Friedman and Rosenman observed in Type A people—those at high risk for coronary artery disease? One popular anecdote about Type A people points us in the right direction. The story is that an upholsterer commented on the chairs he observed in the waiting area of an office building. He noticed that the chairs in this area were worn only on the front edge.

That one visual detail serves up a full-blown image of Type A behavior. We can see people poised on the edge of their seats, glancing nervously at their watches every few seconds, growing more impatient at having to wait, and contemplating how to chew out anyone remotely responsible for delaying a scheduled appointment.

Indeed, Type A people suffer from something Friedman and Rosenman called "hurry sickness." They defined hurry sickness as "an insatiable desire to accomplish too much or to take part in too many events in the amount of time available."

The typical strategies used by Type A people to satisfy this limitless desire are to speed up nearly all daily activities and to do several things at once. These strategies showed up in activities as basic as bathroom behaviors. In a quest to save time, for example, some Type A men stopped shaving with a blade in favor of shaving with an electric razor. Some of these people even used two electric razors so they could shave both sides of the face at once! Others made a practice of shaving, sitting on the toilet, and scanning the morning newspaper—all at the same time.

Other Type A behaviors described by Friedman and Rosenman include the following:

- Insecurity about status—a nagging sense of failure and belief that one's achievements usually fail to match up with someone else's expectations.
- Hyperaggressiveness—a desire not only to win over others but to dominate them.
- Free-floating hostility—a pervasive anger that readily surfaces over trivial events. This anger is the most

critical factor in the Type A's personality, one that can result in devastating health consequences.

- A drive to self-destruction—a covert instinct to make choices that threaten to ruin one's career or personal health.

Friedman and Rosenman contrasted Type A behavior with another approach to life called Type B behavior. In contrast to Type A people, Type B persons are on gracious terms with time. They value themselves as much for what they've already done as for what they can accomplish in the future. Type B people have little desire to control other people, and they have a healthy sense of self-esteem. These people typically take pleasure in viewing art, listening to music, reading, contemplation, and other activities that Type A people see as a waste of time.

This distinction between two types of people is useful. However, I've found it's too easy to talk about Type A people in mostly negative terms. It's true that many people we label Type A seem like they're on a treadmill. Yet some have chosen to be on the treadmill and like being there. The crucial question is: Do people on the treadmill have control of the switch? Can they choose when to turn that switch off and on? Those who can control the switch could be showing healthful levels of commitment toward a goal.

Categorizing people as Type A or Type B is too limiting. There's a more positive way to talk about a healthful approach to life: the Type C person, or the C personality. Why talk about another category? Because in describing wellness I find myself naturally using lots of "C" words. C persons are courageous, creative, comfortable, composed, and confident. C personalities combine the productivity of Type A people with the leisurely outlook of Type B people. In doing so, C personalities create a lifestyle that promotes long-term health.

Healthy people are much like the top-performing athletes Robert Kriegel depicts in his book *C Zone—Peak Performance Under Pressure*. Type C people excel in the biggest game there is—the sport of healthy living. Symphony orchestra conductors are also C personalities, and conduct themselves "well." For me, the primary characteristics of Type C behavior boil down to five C's: being conditioned, connected, challenged, committed, and controlled. We'll look at each of these in turn.

Conditioned

By learning how to J'ARM, you've already explored one aspect of the Type C person: conditioning. Conducting, another one of those "C words", is exercise—that is, physical conditioning. Earlier in this book, especially in Chapter Three, you read about how to carry out this kind of conditioning. From the standpoint of the C personality, however, another kind of conditioning is equally important: mental conditioning.

Mental conditioning becomes especially important as people grow older. To understand why, remember that we really have three distinct ages: a chronological age, a physiological age, and a mental age.

Anyone who still has a birth certificate can verify her chronological age—the number of years and days that person has lived. That's fairly straightforward.

Physiological age is a more subtle concept, however. This age has a lot to do with one's state of health. During the first months of his presidency, former president George Bush underwent a physical examination. He was 65 at the time, but his physician said that he had the physical condition of a man of 55. This fact is not surprising, since we know that Bush is a runner and keeps up a regular exercise regimen. He gives us an example of how physiological age can prevail over chronological age, the inexorable march of passing years. I believe the reason George Bush is so "young" physiologically is that he works and plays at becoming a Type C Personality.

That brings us to the third concept, mental age. Here we could profit from studying the lives of the great comedians—not those who burned out or died young, but those who used humor to keep themselves perennially young at heart. One of my favorite examples was George Burns. Once someone asked him if he had a happy childhood. "So far," was his reply. Another person asked George how it felt to be 85. "When I feel 85," he said, "I'll let you know."

Another person who comes to mind is Satchel Paige, the great baseball player and legendary pitcher. Paige was black, and racial discrimination barred him from the major leagues until relatively late in his career. By the time he joined the Cleveland Indians in 1948, Paige was already older than most of the other players. Add to this the fact that Paige really didn't know his chronological age. No one could remember his exact birth date, and he didn't have a birth certificate. According to some reports, not even Paige's mother, who gave birth to a large family, could remember exactly when Satchel was born.

There grew a kind of mystique about this whole matter. Reporters, awed at Paige's prowess on the baseball field, kept asking him how old he was. Once Paige lost his patience and turned the tables on an inquiring reporter by firing back a single question: "Young man," he asked, "how old would you be if you didn't know how old you was?"

That question is relevant to all of us. It reminds us that we don't have to act according to anyone's preconceived notions about what people are "supposed" to act like at age 60, 70, or 80. Throw away the stereotypes about aging, and discourage the jokes about age that dwell on loss of various mental and bodily functions.

Pretend for a moment that your birth certificate has been lost forever and no one has a clue to the day and year you entered the world. How old do you feel right now? How much energy do you have to accomplish the things that matter? What projects and goals are you actively pursuing? What activities imbue your life with a sense of passion and purpose? Would knowing your chronological age make any difference in all this? Please consider putting on the mental "costume" of a younger age.

These questions bring us to the core of the C personality. Physical conditioning is important; no one denies that. Yet it's easy to gloss over the difference we can make by giving conscious attention to our mental age. The C personality does this by living out the other "significant C's" of life—by staying connected, challenged, committed, and controlled.

Connected

We know that endorphin levels are raised when people spend time with friends and family. A popular word for relating to others is "connecting." As a physician, I know that connecting is important in any type of treatment program for chronic illness. Most people in such treatment improve when they're connected to people at work and at home. Connections to the community, through volunteer activities and political work, are also powerful. So are touching and hugging, our most basic form of connecting. And in their quest for meaning, many find connecting to a spiritual community and a sacred reality to be equally essential.

Even connecting to a pet can have a healing effect. Some research indicates that pet owners who have surgery get out of the hospital faster than those who don't. People who have pets at home want to go home and take care of them. These people feel needed—an excellent argument, I think, for owning pets. In fact, one study indicates that VPS (Vintage People) who own a dog see their physician 16 percent less than people without dogs. It's a little threatening to me as a physician to think that I can be replaced by a dog that percentage of the time! Dogs have been found to be the most healthful pets for several reasons. People frequently exercise with them. They act as counselors because we can talk to them often as we would another person. And we pet and groom them more then other pets. Isn't that "touching"?

Many of the people with chronic aches and pain who come to see me are not well connected. Gertie was an example of that. She had retired and failed to keep ties with former coworkers, and her family lived some distance away. She had no really close friends. She had no church or spiritual connection. She belonged to no clubs nor did she do any community volunteer activities. She lived alone in an apartment with only a television set for company—no pets, no plants.

I suggested that Gertie begin by getting something living in her life by connecting with a pet, perhaps a dog or cat. However, her apartment owner emphatically informed her that no pets were allowed. How about fish? Well, she didn't go for fish. "Then how about plants?" I suggested. "Would you consider raising some plants? After all, those of us who are gardeners know how gratifying this activity is. A hobby such as taking care of a garden can even raise your endorphin levels."

This idea sparked an interest in Gertie, who began by raising some vines and green plants. There were plants all over her apartment. She was supplying plants to others in her building—and meanwhile making new friends. She went to garden shows and garden lectures, growing out of the confines of her solitude.

Gertie was fond of repotting plants, something I told her was an exercise in "plant parenthood." Being part of a "growth industry," she started bringing plants into my office. I still have a plant on my desk, in fact, from Gertie.

After several months I asked her to reflect on her new hobby. "Oh, it's great," she said. "It is challenging. I have something to get up for in the morning. I feel like there is something rooting for me every day. I always wanted to be a plant manager, and now...well, I am one."

Gertie said her favorites were the blooming plants. She went to bed at night and got up in the morning just to look for more blossoms in her apartment. "You know, these plants, all this work that I am putting into them, all this nurturing and this TLC I'm giving them?" she said one day. "Well, when one comes into bloom I can just hear it saying to me, 'Gertie, this bud's for you!'"

A simple living connection with plants was enough to transform Gertie's attitude toward life. The plants helped take Gertie out of herself and share herself again with people and with nature. She had put some "living" in her life. In light of this change, imagine how powerful all connections to friends, family, and a spiritual community can be. Most of us readily acknowledge that fact. At the same time, it's common for people to watch months and even years pass without really connecting to the significant people in their lives. This lack is a hollow at the core of life, a feeling of emptiness, a sense that something is missing. That missing something could be better health.

I suggest you set aside specific times to connect with others, and not just your physician. Treat these times as you would a business appointment or a trip to your beautician or barber. Keep a calendar book and block out times where you plan to do nothing but see friends, eat a quiet, relaxed dinner with your partner, or visit your children or grandchildren. Also set aside times for your spiritual practice, whatever that is. Regular church attendance, prayer, or meditation can greatly increase your sense of being connected.

Challenged

C personalities are those who thrive on challenge. To them, change is not a problem. Change is normal, expected, welcomed, and almost always an opportunity to look for areas of self improvement. These people can even accept defeat as a temporary setback, Often they turn defeat into an opportunity to create new and better circumstances, a chance to learn.and develop new skills.

To some this enthusiasm sounds like wishful thinking or a hollow pep-talk. My only response is, give it a try. Remember that you can talk about any life situation in a way that empowers you. Take these common scenarios:

- "I just found out I owe another $1,000 in income taxes."
- "I just got fired."
- "My lower back aches most of the time."

Here are some common responses to these situations:

- "How terrible. How could I have made such a mistake?"
- "Getting fired is the end of the road. There's no hope for me now."
- "When my back hurts like this, there's nothing I can do."

None of there responses is inevitable. Instead, you could respond in more positive ways:

- "Wow! I owe more in taxes. That probably means I made a lot more money last year. I deserve congratulations." "What a wonderful opportunity, honor and privilege it is to live in the USA and enjoy the quality of life my tax dollars help support."
- "Many other people have survived getting fired and gone on to more satisfying careers. Now I have the time to explore what I really want to do. Then I can get a job that really draws on my interests, one that stimulates and challenges my creativity."
- "Maybe this back pain is a signal that some part of my lifestyle isn't working well. I can find out what lifestyle factors are contributing to my pain and modify them. When I do, I'll be more in charge of my health."

As you can imagine, the second set of responses will lead to far different results than the first set. Just keep in mind that you can choose your response to any event in your life, even when you can't change the event itself. And there are literally thousands of possible responses to any life event.

When you feel threatened by change, search for an attitude that benefits you. Then act on that attitude.

This brings us to the commitment, the next element of the C personality: putting on a pos"I"tive mental costume.

Committed

C persons have a commitment to projects as well as people. They have goals—realistic goals, long-term goals, short-range goals. What's more, they have specific plans for reaching those goals, and they act on their plans with enthusiasm—a word which, by the way, means "God within". You might say these people stop feeling sorry for themselves and get off their duffs. They get ready, they aim, and they fire! They commence and concentrate on their goals. They chart their course. (Notice all those "C words" again.)

What do you really want? Have you taken any time recently to reflect on this question? When people do, they often come up with vague wishes and desires: to be happy, to be fulfilled, to be more creative, more financially secure. Well, fine. But what do those wishes really mean? Exactly what can you do to become more creative, happy, and financially secure? And how will you know whether you're making any progress toward those states of well-being?

A goal that remains hazy and undefined is likely to wither and die. To get around this problem, start to chart the course. Planning does not have to be an arduous task that kills your spontaneity. Instead, it can be a tool for increasing the freedom in your life.

Here's a sure-fire way to make your goals so real that you can almost touch them. Take any goal you'd like to achieve—say, furthering your education. If you were really moving toward this goal, then how would your life be different right now? One possibility is that you'd be taking evening classes at a local college, community education program, or elderhostel. Well, what's needed to make that happen? First you'd want to find out what courses are being offered and which courses are open to people like yourself. You'd also want to find out what these courses cost, when they meet, and who teaches them. One way to answer these questions is to get a course catalog. Now your goal becomes to call or write for a course catalog. By the way, feel free to ask for help at any step. VPS for example, can ask for assistance from senior citizen centers.

All this is simple, common sense. But notice what's happening here. A goal that was unformed and unclear—furthering your education or simply learning more—has been transformed into something as clear and concrete as writing a letter or making a phone call.

That's the key to getting many of the things you want from life. In other words, take your goal and analyze it down to an action you can take today. Make that action so specific that you can write it down on today's "to-do" list. Go through this process as many times as necessary to make your goal a reality.

When you do this, you're planning. That's really all there is to it. Remember that there are two primary reasons people fail to achieve their goals: One, they don't have any clear goals; two, even if they have goals, they don't take the time to make a plan for achieving them. To get past these barriers, put your goals in writing and turn them into specific actions.

Planning—that is, setting and reaching goals—is really just another way of describing commitment. Planning is the "get ready" and the "aim" we all need in our life. Yet too many people just aim and aim. What we can many times do is shorten the aiming process and fire—that is, move into action.

Controlled

A 1981 article in the *Wall Street Journal* announced a new product from a company named Personal Electronics, Inc. This was a new watch equipped with a "speak" button. And the most interesting thing about this watch was its alarm system. When the alarm first went off, it played a minuet. If the wearer ignored this signal, the watch responded five minutes later with a shorter piece of music and a synthesized voice that announced the time and spoke a message: "Please hurry."

Americans have a reputation across the world as the people who hurry. We're known for getting things done, for keeping on schedule, and for measuring our effectiveness by the bottom line, knowing that "time is money." This matter of time is crucial. Many of the factors associated with stress have to do with time. People feel stressed when they can't squeeze enough hours into the day. They often feel driven and ambitious. Some of them find it excruciating to stand in line, stop at traffic lights during rush hour, or endure a short wait in the dentist's office. Many of them feel they just can never get enough time. This feeling is common among Type A personalities. In a real sense, their illnesses are time-driven.

Ask people who feel a constant need to hurry if they feel in control over their lives. Chances are they'll say no. At the root of that feeling is their use of time. A powerful step toward getting in control of your time (and your life) is to manage time wisely. You can begin by keeping track of how you presently use time. Buy an inexpensive appointment book with slots for each hour of the day. For one week, note what you do each hour. Just a simple word or phrase will do: dressing, shaving, sleeping, eating, reading, watching television.

After the week is over, analyze your use of time. How many hours did you spend on each activity? Does your use of time reflect what you feel is truly important? Are there pockets of wasted time in your day, periods that you could put to better use? Do you allow enough time to slow down, relax, read, prepare nutritious meals, and talk to friends and family?

This is a simple yet highly revealing exercise. It's powerful because it gives you something concrete to work with—the facts about how you use time. Armed with this knowledge, you can choose different ways to spend your time. After monitoring your time for one week, practice planning. Decide how you want to use your time. Choose the four or five most important tasks you'd like to accomplish each day. Then block out times for them in your appointment book. Be sure to schedule times for the actions that can lead you to your long- and short-term goals.

Of course, there are many other ways you can increase your sense of control. When you start a task, stay at the job until it is completed. Seeing a project through from beginning to end reinforces a sense of control. Also, continue to learn. Increasing our knowledge and skills makes us more competent. That, in turn, gives us a feeling of control.

Another aspect of control is choice, particularly the choices that affect health. C persons believe that they have some control over their health. We do have a great deal of control over our state of health. Yet, according to some polls, only 26 percent of our population believes that this is true. I'm sure you won't be surprised when I tell you that the healthiest people in our society are often those who believe that they have some control over their health.

This matter of choice and control over health is something

I've worked with all my life. I got into health education because I have a very high cholesterol level. There's a genetic factor at work: All the men in my family have died in their fifties or early sixties with a high cholesterol problem. My cholesterol while I was in medical school was 510.

That has led to some profound changes in my lifestyle. For thirty years I haven't eaten an egg. (Like Jack Spratt, I can eat no fat.) I run, J'ARM, set short- and long-term goals, and consciously make doses of laughter a staple in my life. I look upon life as a game, one that's exhilarating to play, even though I've been dealt a bad card when it comes to cholesterol.

I admit the observation that life is a game doesn't sound very profound. You've heard it before. Yet it's important to specify what kind of a game we're talking about. It's not a roulette game where blind chance and factors beyond your control determine the inevitable outcome. Rather, life is more like a bridge or a poker game, a contest of skill and strategy. The best bridge players don't always get the best hands. Rather, they know how to play the hand that they've been dealt. Simply put, they take control.

Yes, life is a game with many strategies and plays, many ways to score health points. But ultimately it is a game we cannot win. At the final buzzer, however, I hope we can all say we gave it our all. The fun is in the playing of the game, not in the winning.

Making lifestyle choices to promote health puts you in control. And this sense of control goes hand in hand with an honest admission of our limits. All the exercise programs and healthful nutrition in the world won't erase our mortality. Even so, accepting this fact can promote our well being.

I was reminded of this several years ago while I was in training for a long run. Always at about the same spot in my training workout, I would start experiencing some tight chest pain. Of course, with my family history, I was concerned about these symptoms. After a week of indecision, I took a treadmill test, which showed a blood supply abnormality of the heart. Then I had an angiogram, which is an x-ray study of the heart. This test showed that in one of my arteries there was a blockage of about 80 percent.

This discovery lead to my decision to undergo an artery-opening procedure called an angioplasty. During this procedure, a long catheter with a small balloon on one end is guided through a large artery in the groin and threaded into the blocked heart artery. When the balloon is properly positioned it is inflated, and the built-up cholesterol deposit is squeezed back into the wall of the artery. This gives a larger opening and improved blood circulation to the heart muscle. During this procedure, the cardiologist inserted a second long catheter through another groin vessel, this one equipped with a defibrillator tip to be used in case my heart stopped or developed an abnormal beat. The defibrillator sends an electrical impulse to the heart that prompts it to start beating normally again.

During the angioplasty, my heart did stop. My doctor pushed the defibrillator button to shock the heart, and my heart still did not start beating. After 30 seconds, he pushed the button again. Nothing happened. After four tries and 90 seconds, my heart finally started again.

This was a significant event, though I can joke about it now. The cardiologist said that poor blood flow to the brain for over a minute could result in some brain damage. I'm sure my family has been wondering how they will ever be able to tell the difference! My three sons have often groaned at my jokes and can say with some truth that Dad has always been a little "funny."

I didn't have any mystical or "out-of-the-body" experiences during those 90 seconds my heart stopped. But I did re-enter life with a renewed sense of what's truly important. To me, every day is now poignant and full of beauty. I can echo the words of the Psalmist: "This is the day the Lord hath made. Rejoice and be glad in it." I now more poignantly appreciate the beauty and value of nature and those around me and the miracle of my own life.

My friend Rosita Perez has a saying: "Don't sweat the little stuff." I asked her, "What's the big stuff?" "Well, first of all, you're born," says Rosita. "Eventually you die. Everything else is the little stuff." Keeping a constructive sense of our own mortality can cut most of our worries down to size. Most of what we get anxious about is the "little stuff."

An effective thing to ask ourselves in difficult times is this: What difference will this problem make in five years? Is this really "big stuff" or "little stuff"? Such questions are often enough to move a problem from the "tragedy" pile to the "inconvenience" pile. Making that mental move puts us back in control.

CHAPTER

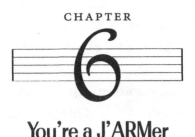

You're a J'ARMer

*Good health is much closer to home, much simpler
(and more enjoyable) than we had imagined.
It derives from a pursuit of healthy pleasures.*
—Robert Ornstein and David Sobel

THIS BOOK HAS TRAVELED A WIDE TERRITORY. EVERYTHING
from endorphins and placebos to conducting yourself to better
health. I'd like to tie it all together with a short summary and a
few words of encouragement.

How to J'ARM: A quick review

If your shoulders are in good shape and you can use your
upper arms, then there's really no wrong way to J'ARM. To
improve the effectiveness of your exercise, however, keep the following points in mind:

- Raise your arms up high, holding a real or imaginary
  conductor's baton. A pen or chopstick makes a great
  baton.

- Play "happy music" that generates pleasant thoughts. If a recording or sound system is not available, then "play" your favorite tunes in your head. J'ARM to your internal music.
- Move your arms vigorously up and down in exaggerated, enthusiastic conductor movements. Sing along with the music.
- Remember that you are the conductor. Allow yourself to feel the music. Stand, dance, or march when you J'ARM to increase the aerobic benefits. You can also J'ARM while you do any repeated movement, such as rising from a sitting to a standing position again and again.
- If possible, look in a mirror while you J'ARM to see yourself as the happy conductor. Freeze this positive image of yourself in your mind. Remind yourself of the benefits of regular exercise, and believe that you can experience those benefits.

The bottom line: Raising a family of pleasure-seeking J'ARMers

J'ARMING and the C personality manifest an outlook on life. What's involved is the big "A" word—attitude. And the central feature of this attitude is that it's OK to seek pleasure. These are not the shallow, one-shot pleasures, like getting drunk or gorging on food, but the deep-seated and enduring pleasures: lifelong friendships, creative work, art, and music. They also find and give healthy pleasures in small doses like a smile, flower, sincere compliment, loving touch, card, or small gift. C personalities also love to give pleasures. But most of all, they expect pleasures. They feel that, simply being alive, they have a right to enjoyment.

This is one of the most profound lessons we can teach our children and grandchildren. It is OK to enjoy ourselves. We can teach our children how to exercise, eat wisely, and make choices that promote a lifetime of health. We can teach them to regularly raise their endorphin levels, to laugh, to enjoy great music. These kinds of pleasures are our birthright. Let us pass them on to our descendants.

Too often we give our children mixed messages about pleasure. We coax babies to giggle and laugh. Then when they get to be toddlers, we start telling them that laughter, smiling, and giggling is not proper: "Don't laugh in church. Don't laugh in school. You're too silly. Act your age. Just grow up!" "Get to work and stop the funny business." "You're supposed to be working, not having fun." What a tragedy that often our society puts down laughter. We put down raising the endorphins.

Children learn attitudes and beliefs the same way they learn a language—by imitation. It has been said that:

> *"No written word or mortal plea can teach young hearts what they should be; nor all the books upon the shelves, but what the teachers are themselves."*

A child born into an Italian home learns the Italian language as well as the body language, culture, feelings, beliefs, and the laughter patterns of these people. The process is similar with children born into a Chinese or a Russian family. That is, children learn by immersion. They absorb not only the spoken word, but the attitudes and temperament of their families.

I implore all parents and grandparents to fill their lives with healthy pleasure. I urge them to immerse their families in laughter and music. Teach optimism by being optimistic. Teach healthy life styles by living a healthy life style—by using seat belts, exercising, avoiding smoking, and eating nutritiously. Teach your children and grandchildren that they are born into an endorphin-raising family where smiling is the most frequent form of communication. Most of all, teach these things by example—even if you have to fake it at times! Teach your children that it doesn't hurt to laugh—that the language called laughter is fluently spoken. Indeed, teach that it is good to laugh just for the health of it.

Satisfaction guaranteed

I've developed and followed my plan to J'ARM for many years. Instead of prescribing an apple a day, I strongly recommend that people J'ARM daily to keep the doctor away. Follow the simple steps outlined in this book and you'll be well on your way to greater conditioning, connection, commitment, challenge, and control in your life. You may not make it to Carnegie Hall to perform as the evening's conductor. However, I guarantee you will have a lot of fun conducting your inner music—an endorphin-raising performance that can get you high on life.

So begin the music, and let's J'ARM We'll have more fun than you can shake a stick at! Remember today's performance is not a dress rehearsal—it's the real thing, the only show in town. Each day begin and end on a high note: J'ARM And may it always be said that you CONDUCTED YOURSELF WELL.

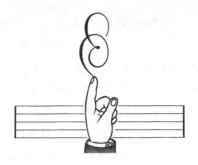

Suggestions for Music

LISTED BELOW ARE SOME RECORDING ARTISTS AND PIECES OF music that I've found useful for J'ARMING. This is not an exhaustive list, only a place to start if you're looking for ideas. Feel free to experiment and add to this list as you find new favorites.

One of the enduring pleasures of life is discovering a piece of music that strikes a personal chord and lifts your spirits. To increase your chances of experiencing that pleasure over and over again, stay open to all kinds of music. If you're a die-hard classical fan, sample some Duke Ellington. If you swear by polkas, get out an a limb and try some Vivaldi. And even if you swoon at the voice of Pavarotti, be willing to put some early Beatles recordings in your music player.

Forget the labels—jazz, classical, rock, country-western, and all the rest. Musicians today, especially "pop" artists, borrow from many styles as they create. The labels we grew up with may no longer yield an accurate map of the musical territory. To keep your J'ARMING program interesting, go for a variety of music.

Keep in mind, too, that music associated with certain occasions or times of the year can be suitable for listening year-round. You can enjoy holiday music anytime, as well as the music played during the central events in your life—weddings, bar mitzvahs, birthdays, and other celebrations.

When you ask people to recommend music that calms and uplifts the spirit, some of them may mention so-called "new age" recordings. Some people I know react negatively to that term, as I did at first. Again, do not let the label scare you away. "New age" is such a broad term that it now encompasses something for just about everyone—everything from Bach to light jazz. If you poke around the "new age" bins in music stores, you may well find something you like. One advantage of doing so is that many of the people interested in creating, recording, and distributing this music are especially interested in the effects of music on the human psyche and body. Their work therefore meshes with the ideas in this book.

I recommend you adopt a daily diet of uplifting music. This regimen is calorie-free. Paired with J'ARMING, the health benefits it yields can last a lifetime. One place to start is with any recordings of simple, upbeat popular songs. These include:

"Smile"
"Put on a Happy Face"
"This Land Is Your Land"
"The Happy Wanderer"
"Hail, Hail the Gang's All Here"
"Oh, What a Beautiful Morning"
"On the Sunny Side Of The Street"
"Happy Days Are Here Again"
"If I Had a Hammer"
"Smiles"
"Keep Young at Heart"
"Mickey Mouse March"
"The More We Get Together"
"Oh When the Saints Go Marching In"

Also J'ARM to music from your favorite cartoons, television shows, and film soundtracks. This could range from *"The Sound of Music"* or *"The Music Man"* to the themes from *"I Love Lucy"* or *"The Dick Van Dyke Show."*

In keeping with the spirit of open-mindedness, the following suggestions are listed alphabetically without regard to category or type of music. Choose what works for you. Many of them are available in cassettes, albums, and compact disks for free from your local library. And of course, there are many, many more.

Bach
Concerto in G Minor for Flute and Strings
Mass in B Minor
Aire on a G-String
The Well-Tempered Clavier

Corelli
Concerto no. 7 in D Minor
Concerto no. 8 in D Minor
Concerto no. 9 in A Major
Concerto no. 10 in F Major

Halpern, Steven
Dawn

Handel
Concerto no. 1 in B-Flat Major
Concerto no. 1 in F
Concerto no. 3 in D

Holst, Gustav
The Planets

Horn, Paul
Inside

Kitaro
Silk Road

Line, Lorie
piano favorites (multiple recordings)

Lynch, Ray
Deep Breakfast
No Blue Thing

Pachabel
Canon in D Major

Stearns, Michael
Morning Jewel

Tchaikovsky
Piano Concerto in B Minor

Telemann
Concerto in G Major

Vivaldi
Concerto in C Major for Mandolin, Strings, and Harpsichord
Concerto in D Major for Guitar and Strings
Concerto in D Minor for Viola d'Amore
Concerto in F Major
The Four Seasons

Windham Hill
See the series of Windham Hill "sampler" recordings, anthologies of recordings by various artists, released annually. These may lead you to individual artists you like.

Winston, George
Autumn

Winter, Paul
Common Ground

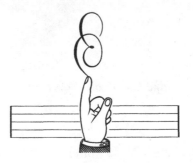

Suggestions for Further Reading

Chesterman, Robert, ed. *Conversations with Conductors,* Totowa, NJ: Rowman and Littlefield, 1976.

Cousins, Norman. *Head First: The Biology of Hope,* New York, NY: Dutton, 1989.

Cousins, Norman. *Anatomy of an Illness as Perceived by the Patient,* New York, NY: Bantam, 1979.

Cousins, Norman. *The Healing Heart: Antidotes to Panic and Helplessness,* New York, NY: Norton, 1983.

Davis, Joel. *Endorphins: New Waves in Brain Chemistry,* Garden City, NY: Dial, 1984.

Friedman, Meyer and Diane Ulmer. *Treating Type A Behavior and Your Heart,* New York, NY: Alfred A. Knopf, 1984.

Halpern, Steven with Louis Savary. *Sound Health: Music and Sounds That Make Us Whole,* San Francisco, CA: Harper and Row, 1985.

Ornstein, Robert and David Sobel. *The Healing Brain,* New York, NY: Simon and Schuster, 1987.

Ornstein, Robert and David Sobel. *Healthy Pleasures,* Reading, MA: Addison-Wesley, 1989.

Padus, Emrika, ed. *The Complete Guide to Your Emotions & Your Health: New Dimensions in Mind/Body Healing,* Emmaus, PA: Rodale Press, 1986.

Waitley, Denis. *The Winner's Edge,* New York, NY: Times Books, 1980.

Ziglar, Zig. *See You at the Top,* Gretna, LA: Pelican, 1979.

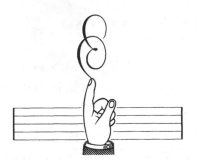

Index

More from Dale Anderson, MD
Available from Chronimed Publishing

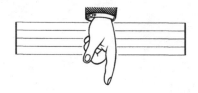

Muscle Pain Relief in 90 Seconds
THE FOLD AND HOLD METHOD

If you suffer from back pain, tennis or golfer's elbow, head or neck pain, wrist pain, shin splints, carpal tunnel syndrome, or any other common muscle pain, Dr. Dale Anderson's innovative "Fold and Hold" Technique can help! "Fold and Hold" combines simple, safe, biomechanical self-treatment with the natural healing powers of the human body. The result is muscle pain relief in 90 seconds.

ISBN 1-56561-058-X • 192 pages • 5½ x 8¾ • paper • **$10.95**

Act Now!
PROVEN ACTING TECHNIQUES YOU CAN USE EVERYDAY TO DRAMATICALLY IMPROVE HEALTH, WEALTH, AND RELATIONSHIPS

Here's a medically proven way to start a dramatic turn of events in your life—from health to relationships to wealth. This innovative guide helps you get in the act by showing how to change your body chemistry through positively scripting, staging, costuming, directing, and acting healthy and happy. The result is often a treatment in itself as well as an effective complement to conventional medications.

ISBN 1-56561-067-9 • 254 pages • 5½ x 8¾ • paper • **$11.95**

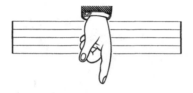

Order by Mail

Chronimed Publishing
P.O. Box 59032
Minneapolis, MN 55459-9686

Place a checkmark next to the book(s) you would like sent. Enclosed is $_____. (Please add $3.00 to this order to cover postage and handling. Minnesota residents add 6.5% sales tax.) Send check or money order—no cash or C.O.D.s. Prices and availability are subject to change without notice.

Name _____

Address _____

City _____ State _____ ZIP _____

— or —

Order by phone—1-800-848-2793
Please have your credit card ready.

Allow 4 to 6 weeks for delivery.
Quantity discounts available upon request.
Prices and availability subject to change without notice.

Source code: TOC

CPSIA information can be obtained
at www.ICGtesting.com
Printed in the USA
JSHW060320130423
40193JS00009BA/455